Lesley Berk MA (Clin Psych) is a psychologist with extensive experience in the clinical management of bipolar and other mood disord.... ⸱⸱ has also been involved in ⸱⸱⸱⸱ research in bipolar disorder and has contributed to scientific journals and presented at conferences in this area.

Michael Berk MBBCh, MMed (Psych), FF(Psych), FRANZCP, PhD is Professor of Psychiatry at Barwon Health and The Geelong Clinic at The University of Melbourne, and heads the Bipolar program at Orygen Research Centre. He is president of the International Society of Bipolar Disorders.

David Castle MB ChB, MSc., MD, DLSHTM, MRCPsych, FRANZCP is Professor of Psychiatry, St Vincent's Health and The University of Melbourne. He has published widely in scientific journals and co-authored 13 books.

Sue Lauder MA (Clin) is a psychologist and has worked in private practice and in a variety of clinical research settings as well as teaching in undergraduate psychology programs. Sue also has a nursing background working in community settings on a range of health and welfare initiatives.

Please visit www.eburypublishing.co.uk/bipolar
to access downloadable forms and other support materials
from the *Living with Bipolar* website.

D0492275

Living with Bipolar

A practical guide for those with the disorder, their family and friends

Lesley Berk, Michael Berk,
David Castle and Sue Lauder

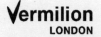

Vermilion
LONDON

1 3 5 7 9 10 8 6 4 2

Published in 2009 by Vermilion, an imprint of Ebury Publishing
First published in Australia by Allen & Unwin in 2008

Ebury Publishing is a Random House Group company

Copyright © Lesley Berk, Michael Berk, David Castle and Sue Lauder 2008

Lesley Berk, Michael Berk, David Castle and Sue Lauder have asserted their right to
be identified as the authors of this Work in accordance with the Copyright, Designs
and Patents Act 1988.

All rights reserved. No part of this publication may be reproduced, stored in
a retrieval system, or transmitted in any form or by any means, electronic,
mechanical, photocopying, recording or otherwise, without the prior permission
of the copyright owner.

The Random House Group Limited Reg. No. 954009

Addresses for companies within the Random House Group can be found at
www.rbooks.co.uk

A CIP catalogue record for this book is available from the British Library

The Random House Group Limited supports The Forest Stewardship
Council (FSC), the leading international forest certification organisation.
All our titles that are printed on Greenpeace approved FSC certified paper
carry the FSC logo. Our paper procurement policy can be found at
www.rbooks.co.uk/environment

Printed in the UK by CPI Mackays, Chatham, ME5 8TD

ISBN 9780091924256

Copies are available at special rates for bulk orders.
Contact the sales development team on 020 7840 8487 for more information.

To buy books by your favourite authors and register for offers, visit:
www.rbooks.co.uk

The information in this book has been compiled by way of general guidance in
relation to the specific subjects addressed, but is not a substitute and not to be
relied on for medical, healthcare, pharmaceutical or other professional advice on
specific circumstances and in specific locations. Please consult your GP before
changing, stopping or starting any medical treatment. So far as the author is
aware the information given is correct and up to date as at October 2008.
Practice, laws and regulations all change, and the reader should obtain up to date
professional advice on any such issues. The author and publishers disclaim, as
far as the law allows, any liability arising directly or indirectly from the use, or
misuse, of the information contained in this book.

This book is dedicated to those people with bipolar disorder who have touched us with their suffering, taught us with their experiences, inspired us with their resilience, and motivated us to try to make a difference.

CONTENTS

ACKNOWLEDGEMENTS

We want to thank supportive organisations that have facilitated our learning and research with regard to the adjunctive psycho-social treatment of bipolar disorder. These include: Beyond Blue, MBF, Barwon Health, the Geelong Clinic, the Geelong Mood Support Group, Pathways, the Melbourne Clinic, University of Melbourne and the Collaborative Therapy Unit at MHRI. In particular, we thank Monica Gilbert, Neil Cole, Reid Maxwell and Krista Staarup. Special thanks also go to Tania Lewis for her constructive feedback regarding this book.

AUTHORS' NOTE

Names of people with bipolar disorder and their families have been changed to protect their identity.

TABLES
AND
FIGURES

Introduction

This book aims to provide practical information about managing bipolar disorder for people with bipolar disorder and those close to them—their partners, close relatives and friends. The idea of writing a book came from people with bipolar disorder in our treatment programs, who requested more information about their illness and its treatment. They wanted information that combined the latest research with practical, hands-on suggestions relevant to their daily lives. This information was requested not only for themselves, but also for the people important to them, to help them understand and find ways of dealing with bipolar disorder. The information we present here comes from current research findings, our clinical experience and from those people with bipolar disorder who have taught us so much about helpful strategies for living with their illness.

Bipolar disorder, previously referred to as manic depression, is about mood swings, but they are no ordinary mood swings. If you have bipolar disorder, you will know that rather than simply experiencing the usual ups and downs of everyday life, you can experience extreme highs and lows that seem to take on a life of their own independent of events around you. You may experience different degrees of these mood states, ranging from hardly noticeable to very severe at different times. You may also have some aspects of high mood combined with low mood at the same time.

These mood swings are *not* character flaws. They result from biological changes in areas of the brain that control mood. These biological changes respond to medication, and bipolar disorder is considered to be an illness. The illness does not end when your extreme mood subsides—rather, it is a recurrent illness that may be compared to asthma. People with asthma experience recurrent attacks, and different degrees of wellness between attacks. The thing about the 'attacks' in bipolar disorder is that they are so personal. They bring about changes in how you feel, both physically and emotionally, in what you think and what you do. Some of these changes can have serious consequences for your safety, and affect your finances, your career and relationships. Fortunately, there *are* effective treatments and personal strategies for managing episodes and preventing relapse.

We include information about bipolar disorder, its causes and triggers, treatment options and ways of preventing relapse, minimising possible negative consequences and dealing with the impact of the illness on your life. Everyone finds some way of coping with their illness, but not all strategies are constructive. This book points out some of the common pitfalls that can be unhelpful or make your illness worse, as well as strategies that help. In addition, we try to address some of the questions we have encountered from patients and their families over the years. We examine ways of keeping an eye on your bipolar disorder, implementing healthy lifestyle choices and drawing up your own relapse prevention plans. You can combine this information with your personal experience and discover new ideas for managing your illness, or confirm your own successful strategies.

The strategies for managing bipolar disorder mentioned here are not intended to replace your medical or psychological treatment. They aim to assist you to be informed, get the best from your treatment and augment it with your own personal strategies.

Finding personal strategies for managing your illness has been termed 'self-management' (Russell, 2005). Sarah Russell, a researcher who has interviewed people about their experience of dealing with bipolar disorder, explains how misleading this term can be. It can seem to indicate that people manage all alone. What self-management of bipolar disorder really means is using the resources available to you for managing your illness wisely. Your bipolar disorder often affects those close to you, some of whom might have little understanding of the illness, or of how they could help. Here we provide information to assist those who care about you in dealing with bipolar disorder. We discuss ways of involving trusted others in the management of your illness, and of enhancing your relationship with your clinician. Bipolar disorder is potentially a very isolating and challenging illness, and having allies in your battle to manage it is a distinct advantage. Enjoying good relationships is part of the richness of life, and we emphasise the importance of finding people you can relate to and of maintaining good relationships.

Living with bipolar disorder also involves adapting to the changes the illness brings to your life. We have found that people who live well with their bipolar disorder combine living a healthy lifestyle with constructive plans for managing the different phases of their illness.

Bipolar disorder is an illness that can affect your life and who you are to the point that the boundary between you and the illness blurs. There may be times when you are so ill that all your energy is devoted to battling your illness and simply surviving. When you are well you may still need to take prescribed medications and keep an eye on your disorder, or attend to a few mild persistent symptoms, but it is easier to devote more attention to the things in life that matter to you, your own goals and interests. Many people report that the illness never leaves them, but it can become a smaller and smaller part of whom they are. Being well provides the opportunity to rebuild your life and yourself. We examine ways of keeping well and enriching life.

The suffering and negative consequences experienced at times as a result of the illness must not be underplayed. At the same time, having bipolar disorder has been connected with creativity, achievement and fame. People like the artist Vincent Van Gogh, composer Robert Schumann and author Virginia Woolf all had bipolar disorder. Bipolar disorder is quite common and affects the lives of many ordinary people. Over one in every hundred people has the diagnosis of bipolar disorder and you can add another two to four people in a hundred if you consider its milder forms as well. The disorder affects women and men equally, as it does people in different countries and from different socioeconomic levels. Despite its prevalence, however, bipolar disorder is not yet completely understood. An added burden for people with bipolar disorder is that unlike illnesses such as asthma, bipolar disorder carries the stigma of 'mental illness', which makes it harder for many people to accept. We discuss ways of coming to terms with your illness and living beyond the confines of stigma.

It can take time to develop a fulfilling lifestyle that helps you keep well. There may still be times when your symptoms break through and you need to use your personal strategies for preventing or minimising relapse. It helps to be prepared. This book aims to demystify the illness, enhance understanding and acceptance and provide practical options for your own strategies. We see managing your bipolar disorder as part of the larger journey of living your life, and hope that this book provides you with ideas and inspiration along the way.

1 WHAT IS BIPOLAR DISORDER?

Being diagnosed with bipolar disorder meant that finally not only did my moods have a name but there was also something I could do to get them more under control. This name did not capture all my experience and the impact that bipolar disorder had on my life but it provided an explanation and a way forward. **Phillip**

Bipolar disorder involves biological changes in mood that are more noticeable, severe, longer lasting and often more disruptive than everyday ups and downs. Recognition of the difficulties and the burdens experienced by people with these extreme mood swings intensified the search for a common language to help describe and treat bipolar disorder. The typical mood changes that occur in the disorder have been organised into specific categories to make them easier to understand, diagnose and treat. In this chapter we discuss the current classification of bipolar disorder. People with bipolar disorder experience the illness differently depending on their symptoms, how often they occur and how their lives are affected. Knowing the current classifications and how they apply to your own experience may assist you in managing your illness.

It is also helpful to be aware of and to recognise symptoms from other disorders, such as drug and alcohol abuse and anxiety, that may be causing additional distress. As we find out more about bipolar disorder, the current diagnostic system may be refined to include milder manifestations of the illness and take into account areas of overlap with other mood disorders.

A BIT OF HISTORY

Bipolar disorder is not a new illness. In ancient Greece, people were aware of melancholia (depression) and mania. In 1851, the French psychiatrist Jean-Pierre Falret described bipolar disorder as *la folie circulaire*, involving changes from mania to melancholia, and in 1854 neurologist Jules Baillarger described these changes as two different stages of the same illness (*folie à double forme*). Towards the end of that century, the German psychiatrist Emil Kraepelin distinguished schizophrenia, which involves psychotic symptoms such as delusions and hallucinations without the extreme mood symptoms, from manic depression. Much later, in 1979, Karl Leonhard separated bipolar disorder from unipolar depression, which is the experience of depression with no mania or hypomania, and so the idea of 'bipolar disorder' was conceptualised (Goodwin & Redfield Jamison, 2007).

THE DIAGNOSIS OF BIPOLAR DISORDER

Unlike physical illnesses such as diabetes and stroke, bipolar disorder cannot be diagnosed by a medical test such as a blood test or brain scan. Instead, diagnosis relies on identifying your current and past symptoms. The *Diagnostic and Statistical Manual of Mental Disorders* (DSM-IV) (American Psychiatric Association, 2000) and the *International Classification of Diseases* (ICD-10)

(World Health Organisation, 2006) stipulate certain criteria as a guide for diagnosis.

This illness usually starts in adolescence or the early twenties, but can occur later or in earlier childhood where it can present a little differently (see the website attached to this book for resources on bipolar in childhood). Many people report that it took a long time for their bipolar disorder to be correctly diagnosed and treated.

Episodes of illness

Bipolar disorder involves 'episodes' of illness. For a diagnosis of bipolar disorder to be made, you will have experienced an episode of mania or hypomania, or a mixed episode, at some stage in your life. Most people experience depressive episodes and milder forms of depression. Episodes differ in severity, occur when you are acutely ill, and exhibit a number of symptoms over a specific period. Once you have experienced an episode of bipolar disorder, the chances of having another episode are high, but ongoing treatment can help to prevent relapse.

An episode of major depression

A depressive episode occurs when you experience depressive symptoms for at least two weeks that cause you distress and affect your relationships, work or daily activities. According to DSM-IV classification, an episode of depression is diagnosed when you have *five or more* of the symptoms listed below. At least one of these symptoms is:

- depressed mood, which may include intense sadness, emptiness, tearfulness or irritability, or
- a loss of interest or pleasure in things, which lasts nearly all day, nearly every day.

The other possible symptoms include:

- lack of energy, and constant tiredness

- restlessness or alternatively a marked lack of activity, known as *lethargy*, which is noticeable by others
- noticeable changes in appetite and weight, either up or down
- sleep problems, which might involve difficulty in falling asleep, waking up a lot during the night, or waking up early in the morning and being unable to return to sleep; or equally, sleeping too much
- feelings of worthlessness and excessive guilt
- difficulty in concentration and/or poor memory or difficulties in making decisions
- persistent thoughts about death and suicide or hopelessness.

Some people have *psychotic symptoms* as part of their depression. This can include delusions (strong beliefs that have no connection with reality) and/or hallucinations (seeing, hearing or smelling things that are not actually there).

An episode of mania

According to the DSM-IV classification, an episode of mania is diagnosed when your mood is excessively happy, elevated, or irritable for at least a week *or* has led to your being admitted to hospital. *At least three* of the following symptoms (*four* if the mood is irritable) must be present:

- needing less sleep than usual
- thoughts racing so quickly that you may get confused and find it difficult to articulate what you want to say
- talking much more than usual or feeling a pressure to keep talking
- being easily distracted from tasks to attend to irrelevant or unimportant things
- feeling a marked increase in self-esteem or thinking you have unique gifts or talents that you do not have
- increasing activity directed to achieving goals (at work, school or sexually) or increasing restlessness and agitation

- participating excessively in pleasurable activities with no regard for the consequences, for example, massive buying sprees, gambling, irresponsible investments, high sex drive and sexual indiscretions.

Mania is diagnosed if these symptoms are severe enough to cause serious disruption to your work or social activities. As with depression, mania may include the presence of psychotic symptoms, including hallucinations and delusions, related to your mood. Extremely disordered or confused thinking is another psychotic symptom that can occur in mania.

Hypomania

The diagnosis of hypomania is based on similar symptom criteria as mania, except that hypomania is milder or briefer. Although you have symptoms, they are not necessarily disruptive and you may be able to carry out your normal day-to-day activities. Still, the changes in your behaviour are obvious enough to be noticed by others. To be classified as a hypomanic episode, the symptoms must last for at least four days. Hypomania does not involve psychotic symptoms.

Mixed episode

You may have thought that having bipolar disorder means that you experience either the lows or the highs, but many people experience a simultaneous mix of these two opposite poles. At first glance this makes no sense, like being hot and cold or black and white at the same time. However, it is possible to have some symptoms of mania and some of depression at the same time. Recognising this combination is vital, as it has specific implications for your treatment. This is explained in more detail in chapter 7 on medications.

According to the DSM-IV classification, a mixed episode occurs when you have a manic and a depressive episode at the same time for *at least a week* and the symptoms cause significant disruption to your daily life, sometimes necessitating hospitalisation. For example, you experience rapid mood swings (happy, sad, irritable), you need less sleep, your appetite is affected, and you are restless and uptight, undertake risky activities, and may have delusions of excessive unrealistic guilt and suicidal thinking.

Other classifications of mixed states do not require that you have full manic and depressive episodes at the same time (Benazzi, 2007; Cassidy et al., 2007). It is common for people who are depressed to have a few manic symptoms, such as racing thoughts, restlessness or a decreased need for sleep, and for people who are manic to experience isolated symptoms of depression, irritability or suicidal thoughts. Mixed states may be divided into depressive and manic mixed states, depending on which type of symptoms predominate. Marcel, a patient of ours, describes his experience of mixed states:

> During these patches, I am miserable and agitated. I feel impatient, and am so irritable and angry I am scared of what I could do. The way I feel switches from moment to moment. My thoughts are churning like a washing machine. I am very negative, and thoughts of suicide keep intruding. I have harmed myself before when I feel like this. I am restless, feel as though I have to do stuff and keep moving, although I get very disorganised. I can't sleep.

Although some people are just prone to mixed states, in other people illicit drug use may have a role in developing mixed states. For some people, certain antidepressants may exacerbate mixed states.

People with mixed states are more vulnerable to developing symptoms of psychosis, such as hearing voices or having paranoid ideas. As in depressive episodes, there is an increased risk of suicidal ideas and attempts in mixed episodes. Ways of managing this risk are discussed in chapter 13.

TYPES OF BIPOLAR DISORDER

People experience different patterns of episodes which characterise their specific type of bipolar disorder. The dominant patterns outlined in DSM-IV are bipolar I and bipolar II disorder; other categories are cyclothymic disorder, and bipolar disorder not otherwise specified (NOS). These patterns may occur with or without other features, such as rapid cycling or psychotic symptoms. The severity of symptoms varies widely between individuals and in the same person over time.

Bipolar I disorder

This type of bipolar disorder is diagnosed if you have had one or more full manic or mixed episode(s), although you may have had depressive episodes as well, as shown in figure 1.1. Although less common, some people experience episodes of mania without ever experiencing a depressive episode.

Mary, who has bipolar I disorder, describes her experience:

> I was hospitalised five years ago after a manic episode. It was a scary experience for all of us. I did not think there was anything wrong with me but I was behaving so

Figure 1.1 Bipolar I disorder

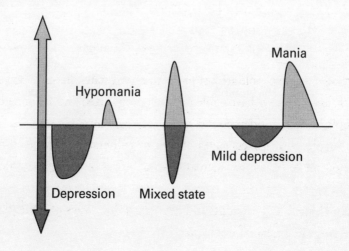

7

strangely, speaking very fast and increasingly incoherently, spending money we did not have, staying up all night and going to parties on my own and inviting people to join my 'grand' schemes, that my husband took me to the doctor. I had married the man of my dreams and we had just had a beautiful baby daughter. The diagnosis of bipolar I disorder sounded cold and clinical and definitely had nothing to do with me. In the next few years I was again hospitalised a few times for mania and once because I was feeling very depressed and suicidal. I have been quite well now for two years and what has helped has been getting to know this illness rather than running away from it. As with any other illness, medication helps, and I have found other strategies that work for me.

Bipolar II disorder

This type involves one or more episodes of hypomania and one or more episodes of depression, but no mania, as illustrated in figure 1.2. If you have bipolar II disorder, you may find that you experience depression more often than hypomania.

Figure 1.2 Bipolar II disorder

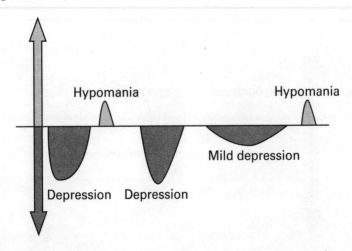

8

Grant discovered he had bipolar II disorder about ten years after his first episode of depression. He explains:

> When I think back, I realise that for years I have had distinct patches lasting a few weeks when I feel much more confident than usual, think and do things more quickly, and have new ideas and goals. I don't need much sleep and instead I get so much done. At this time, my social life peaks and my family remark about my 'unusual energy'. Everything is in techni-colour. Then there are months when things are more grey and sombre and I feel empty and exhausted. Nothing is enjoyable and eventually it becomes a struggle even to get out of bed. For a long time these dark depressions dominated my life. My previous doctor never enquired about my technicolour patches, and they were not disturbing, so I never mentioned them. Recently [my current] doctor asked me about hypo-mania and we discussed changing my treatment.

Cyclothymic disorder

Cyclothymia refers to a pattern involving hypomanic and mild depressive symptoms that have been experienced for two or more

Figure 1.3 Cyclothymic disorder

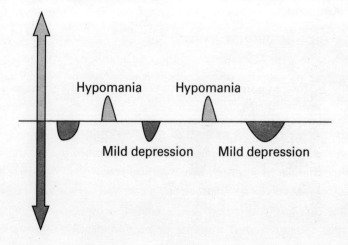

years. Although milder than bipolar I or II, the symptoms of cyclothymic disorder are still severe enough to cause difficulties at work, in education, employment and relationships. Bipolar disorder and cyclothymia exist on a continuum.

Bipolar disorder not otherwise specified

Bipolar disorder NOS is used to diagnose illness episodes that do not last long enough to be described as manic, hypomanic, mixed or major depressive episodes, or which do not have the required number of symptoms.

There is some debate about whether to categorise particular temperaments as bipolar disorder NOS, or to subdivide bipolar disorder further on a continuum from its more severe to its milder presentations. Some people may have temperaments that look like very mild bipolar symptoms and which sometimes later develop into more established forms of bipolar disorder (Akiskal et al., 1998).

- *hyperthymic*: very cheerful, optimistic, extroverted, confident, always busy
- *cyclothymic*: fluctuating mild mood changes, changing levels of self-esteem
- *dysthymic*: usually joyless, lacking energy but not as severe as depression
- *depressive mixed*: mild symptoms of anxiety, irritability, restlessness, sadness.

The bipolar spectrum

For people who have never experienced mania or hypomania, a diagnosis of unipolar illness may be clear. Many people view bipolar disorder as distinct from unipolar disorder. In reality, the difference is less clear-cut. For example, you may have predominant symptoms of depression as well as minor experiences of mood elevation that are too mild or brief to be diagnosed as having bipolar disorder. These symptoms fall into the bipolar spectrum, however, and you may find that you benefit from treatments that are usually used for bipolar disorder. Similarly, some people diagnosed with unipolar depression develop hypomania when taking antidepressant treatment. The boundaries of the spectrum are controversial, but it is likely that almost half of all people who experience diagnosed depression have some form of bipolar disorder. People whose illness falls into the bipolar spectrum are more likely to have depression associated with increased sleep and marked fatigue, and to experience feelings of flatness, rather than sadness.

RAPID CYCLING

Cycling occurs when you swing from one episode of illness, such as depression, into another, such as mania or a mixed state. According to DSM-IV, rapid cycling occurs when you have at least four episodes of illness, either mania or depression, in a calendar year—but rapid cycling can be far more frequent than that, with some people cycling within weeks or even days. Rapid cycling is not rare, occurring in somewhere between 15 and 25 per cent of people who suffer from bipolar disorder. The treatment for people who have a pattern of rapid cycling differs significantly from the treatment for people who don't, so it is important to recognise if this is your pattern.

People who suffer from rapid cycling are more likely to be female and younger, or to have become ill later in life, and may have more episodes and hospitalisations. Thyroid problems and antidepressants may contribute to rapid cycling. For some people, although they cycle from depression to mania, the dominant experience is depression.

SEASONAL PATTERN

Some people find that they usually have episodes at a particular time of year. You may find that you tend to develop a major depressive episode in winter or autumn and/or a hypomanic or manic episode in spring or summer. Knowing these patterns can be useful as you can find ways of preventing or reducing the severity of the episode.

WHAT BIPOLAR DISORDER IS NOT

Bipolar disorder may need to be distinguished from signs and symptoms that resemble it in order for people to get the right treatment. Not all mood swings are bipolar. Most people will experience better or worse days. At times, these can happen in response to the ups and downs of life, but sometimes you can just 'get out of bed on the wrong side'. Mood swings that are within the realm of everyone's experience, such as understandable reactions to an unfortunate event or that are not particularly intense, distressing, disruptive or noticeable, are unlikely to be part of bipolar disorder.

Hypomanic, manic or mixed episodes distinguish bipolar disorder from unipolar depression. Bipolar disorder can also be confused with illnesses that involve psychosis, such as schizophrenia. Schizophrenia involves periods of prominent psychotic symptoms, including delusions, hallucinations and disordered thinking but, rather than experiencing intense moods, schizophrenia is associated with blunted moods. While people with schizophrenia may become depressed, their psychotic symptoms do not occur only in the presence of a manic, hypomanic or depressed episode, as they do in bipolar disorder.

Bipolar disorder has also been confused with schizoaffective disorder, another illness that includes both psychotic and mood symptoms. The essential difference here is that in bipolar disorder psychotic symptoms occur only in the presence of mood symptoms, whereas in schizoaffective disorder psychotic symptoms occur both in the presence of mood symptoms and when mood symptoms have been absent for at least two weeks.

Mood swings are common in borderline personality disorder, but these do not usually last as long and are not as marked as the moods in bipolar disorder. In borderline personality, mood swings occur as a reaction to events and are linked to particular personality characteristics.

Some altered states brought on temporarily by taking certain illicit drugs may mimic episodes of bipolar disorder, but the effects of intoxication wear off rapidly and do not constitute bipolar disorder. The symptoms of certain medical conditions such as hypothyroidism or multiple sclerosis can also mimic bipolar disorder. Accurate diagnosis of bipolar disorder is essential for appropriate treatment.

COMORBIDITY

Bipolar disorder can occur together with many other disorders, so you may find that you have other symptoms besides those of bipolar disorder. This is called 'comorbidity'. Two problems that commonly occur with bipolar disorder are drug and alcohol problems and anxiety.

Alcohol and drug problems

While some people with bipolar disorder have no alcohol or drug problems, there are many (50 to 70 per cent of people with bipolar disorder) whose lives are complicated by these additional difficulties (Brady & Sonne, 1995). Of the substances that are used, by far the most common is alcohol, although there are also high rates of marijuana, cocaine, amphetamine, benzodiazapine and heroin use among people with bipolar disorder. The risk of relapse, mixed episodes, rapid cycling, suicide and violent behaviour are increased in people with bipolar disorder who have drug or alcohol problems (Balázs et al., 2006), thus people with drug or alcohol problems tend to suffer more as they end up more ill, being hospitalised more often, and suffering greater disruption to their lives than people with bipolar disorder who do not abuse these substances.

Facing up to drug and alcohol problems can make an enormous difference to your bipolar disorder and your life. Some people find it hard to reduce their drug or alcohol use even when they know it is causing major problems and undermining their health. If this is your experience, discussing this problem with your clinician may be a first step towards treatment. Remember you are not alone with this dilemma. We list some resources on the website (www.eburypublishing.co.uk/bipolar) that you can use to help reduce your drug or alcohol consumption.

Anxiety

Many people with bipolar disorder experience anxiety, which may be most common in people with bipolar II disorder and in females (McIntyre et al., 2006). Anxiety may predate your bipolar disorder, occur when you experience an episode of bipolar disorder, be part of your rapid cycling or be present when you are well. For some people, anxiety increases the risk of recurrence of bipolar episodes. Anxiety symptoms can be distressing and disruptive, and people with bipolar disorder are becoming increasingly aware of the need to identify and treat their anxiety together with their bipolar disorder. A few helpful resources are listed on the website associated with this book. Many people work at reducing their anxiety together with their clinician.

Your experience of anxiety may range from a few mild symptoms to a disabling disorder. Some anxiety symptoms resemble symptoms of physical illness so it is important to differentiate them. Common anxiety symptoms include:

- increased heart rate, pounding or palpitations
- feeling as if you are short of breath or suffering a choking sensation
- sweating
- feeling dizzy or light-headed or cut off or distant from things
- shaking or trembling
- difficulty concentrating
- nausea, vomiting or diarrhoea
- pins and needles or numbness
- feeling very cold or hot flushes
- aches and pains

- indigestion
- excessive worry
- intense fear of losing control or feelings of dread.

Some people experience anxiety disorders such as panic disorder, specific phobia, social phobia, obsessive-compulsive disorder, post-traumatic stress disorder and generalised anxiety disorder, which are outlined below. Discussing your anxiety problems with your clinician may help you to get the best treatment.

Panic disorder with or without agoraphobia
Panic disorder involves panic attacks, which are short, intense periods of anxiety. Agoraphobia involves anxiety about being in certain situations that feel unsafe and so are avoided, such as being away from home, or in a crowd. For some people, panic attacks are linked to these specific situations.

Specific phobia
Specific phobia involves excessive and irrational anxiety and avoidance of specific objects or events such as snakes, spiders or flying.

Social phobia
Social phobia involves excessive anxiety about how you will perform in social situations and how others will judge you. You may find that you avoid certain social situations, and that even anticipating these situations makes you panic or feel distressed.

Obsessive-compulsive disorder
Obsessions are persistent, intrusive thoughts, impulses or images that cause distress but are hard to stop or ignore. Compulsions are repetitive actions considered to bring relief or prevent disaster related to your obsessions, such as excessively washing your hands, checking things or counting. These obsessions and compulsions can be very time-consuming and disrupt your daily life.

Post-traumatic stress disorder
Post-traumatic stress disorder sometimes occurs when you have experienced a very threatening or traumatic event which evoked

intense fear and helplessness. The event is re-experienced in different ways such as flashbacks, when you encounter things that remind you of the trauma, or in nightmares. As a result you may avoid any associations with or reminders of the event, and generally cut off your feelings. You may feel very distressed, and this can interfere with your daily life.

Generalised anxiety disorder

The predominant symptoms of generalised anxiety disorder are excessive worry and anxiety combined with other symptoms such as difficulty concentrating, sleep disturbances, feeling on edge and unsettled, or fatigued. This anxiety usually persists longer than six months, makes you feel distressed and can interfere with your daily functioning.

KEY POINTS

- Bipolar disorder may be a relatively new name, but this illness was observed even in ancient Greece.
- Having a common language to diagnose and describe bipolar disorder is useful for the management of your illness.
- Bipolar disorder includes a spectrum of different manifestations between classical bipolar disorder and depression as well as milder manifestations of the illness.
- It is important for bipolar disorder to be distinguished from other illnesses so that you can receive the correct treatment. Typically, bipolar disorder can be confused with unipolar depression or schizophrenia.
- Sometimes bipolar disorder can be complicated by symptoms of other disorders. Recognising and treating those symptoms may reduce their impact on your bipolar disorder and your life.
- Combining theoretical knowledge of bipolar disorder with your own insights into your experience of this illness can help you to understand your illness and find appropriate strategies for managing it.

2 BIPOLAR DEPRESSION

My depression was so strange . . . As if the elves had stolen me and had left a block of wood instead.

Marc De Hert et al., *Anything or Nothing*, 2004: 15.

Bipolar depression is not just feeling a bit blue because of the everyday stresses and strains of life. The experience of depression is markedly more distressing and long lasting than that, and can interfere with your daily life and what is important to you. Your mood involves the way you think, feel and behave, as well as the biological changes happening in your brain. In this chapter we look more closely at some of the changes in feelings, thinking and behaviour reported by people with bipolar depression. This depression can be experienced in a variety of ways, depending on the combination of symptoms, their level of severity and how often you experience them. If you recognise your experience in these pages, know that you are not alone. About 90 per cent of people with bipolar disorder experience depression at some time. Although depression may seem endless and overwhelming at times, a lot can be done to treat it and we discuss this in more detail in later chapters. Depression is *not* something you *are*, it is something you *have*. It is not your fault any more than having an illness like asthma is your fault. Getting to know your experience of depression and recognising symptoms as they occur may give you the chance to implement appropriate treatment and strategies early.

WHAT CHANGES WHEN YOU BECOME DEPRESSED?

Below we list a few changes in feeling, thinking and behaving reported by people who have experienced bipolar depression. You may find that you or those close to you have experienced some of these changes.

Changes in feeling

Changes in how you feel include:

No feeling or tears

Many people with bipolar disorder experience an absence of feeling, or feel flat and empty, as part of their depression. For some there is a pervasive feeling of sadness and tearfulness.

Don't care

You sometimes hear people who are feeling depressed declaring that they no longer care about anything, even those things that used to matter to them.

Nothing's interesting

You may lose interest and motivation to do things. Sometimes people don't feel better even temporarily when something good happens.

Can't enjoy anything

You may find that your capacity to experience pleasure diminishes. Many people find their sex drive decreases. Your senses may even be dulled so that things don't taste or smell as good as they used to and the world looks grey.

Too tired, no energy
It is common to feel as though you have just run a marathon and have no energy left.

Mornings are worse
You may feel worse at a particular time of day, especially in the morning, although some people feel worse in the evening.

Worthless
An important clue is a fall in self-esteem, which makes people lack confidence and feel useless, and temporarily forget all their strengths and abilities.

Guilt
You may feel excessively guilty for even minor mistakes or indiscretions, and recall with shame simple, very human errors.

Criticism and rejection
Many people become more sensitive to criticism and rejection.

Irritable, impatient, aggressive
Being more aggressive, argumentative, impatient and irritable in general, or with those closest to you, is common when experiencing depression, mania or mixed states.

Hopeless, helpless
Another clue to recognising depression is the hopelessness you may feel about the future, and the helplessness about not feeling able to change things. When severe, this hopelessness contributes to feeling suicidal.

Worried, anxious
This worry may be a global anxiety when everything is a worry, or limited to something specific, such as worrying about physical health.

Physical symptoms of anxiety
Common anxiety symptoms include tremor, sweating, a racing heart, hot or cold flushes, or discomfort in the stomach or chest.

Aches and pains
Some people experience numerous physical aches and pains when depressed. A warning sign of depression might be an increase in physical symptoms and an increase in trips to the doctor by a person who is generally healthy.

Depressed activity
You may notice changes in what you do including:

Hibernation
Depression has been compared to a kind of hibernation from the world. Even the most outgoing of people may find that when they become depressed they start refusing invitations and want to be alone.

Lethargy
Lethargy means being very tired, unmotivated and slowed down. Joe explains:

> I told him that doing the dishes when I felt like this was similar to him trying to run a race when his body was rendered weak by a fever. He could not see my illness, but it was sapping my energy and making all those tasks one normally takes for granted into major hurdles.

People with bipolar depression may talk slowly, use shorter sentences and move slowly. Outsiders sometimes comment that people who are depressed have fewer facial expressions and gestures. In its milder form, this drop in activity level can mean that it is harder than usual to keep to arrangements or to get going in the morning. Thoughts can become slower and fewer. Lethargy in its more severe form can mean that it is difficult to get even basic things done, or even to get out of bed.

Agitation

Some people experience agitation as part of their depression, so that they find it hard to sit still and are restless. In some cases they may experience fluctuations from being slowed down to being agitated. Agitation can also make it hard to complete tasks.

Procrastination, withdrawal and avoidance

Delaying tasks, withdrawing from commitments or arrangements and avoiding social contacts can all be signs of growing depression.

Sleeping and eating

Depression can affect basic activities such as sleeping and eating. Sleeping much more than usual is typically associated with bipolar depression, although some people with bipolar disorder suffer from insomnia as a sign of depression. Some people with bipolar depression lose their appetite when depressed, resulting in significant weight loss, whereas others crave 'comfort food' and eat more.

Depressed thinking

Your thinking may become more one-sided and negative. Concentration and memory difficulties can temporarily detract from your usual sharpness and slow you down.

Thinking negatively

> The voice of depression is often a bully and it tends to block out alternatives . . . Depression is very keen to tell us what we can't do, what we shouldn't do and how bad things are . . . there are two basic orientations that we can take that will help control it: insisting on rational questioning and alternatives, and developing basic compassion (Gilbert, 2000:99).

In everyday life, even when in a relatively stable mood, everyone experiences negative thoughts from time to time—but depression involves more than occasional negative thinking. It is as if you put on dark glasses and see yourself, others and the future in only one rigid way, the worst and most critical way. Distrustful thoughts or believing that others are against you is also typical of depression— for example, in a stable loving relationship suddenly deciding that your partner is rejecting you or having an affair.

A one-sided, negative interpretation of events is often unrealistically applied to everything and to all time—for example, 'I did not manage to pass this exam so I will never be able to pass an exam or do anything else that is important to me ever again.' Such thinking can increase feelings of hopelessness, so that it's not surprising that people who experience depression may be plagued with thoughts about suicide. Suicidal thoughts need to be taken seriously, because there is a high risk of suicide. Fortunately, there is a lot that can be done to reduce this risk, as explained in chapter 13.

Your thinking may become dominated by selective negative memories from the past or worries about the present or the future. These thoughts sometimes repeat themselves endlessly, so that it is difficult to think of other things. This is called 'rumination'. Cognitive behaviour therapy (CBT) and mindfulness-based psychotherapy both have special strategies that people have found helpful in dealing with depressed thinking (see chapters 8 and 12).

Sluggish thoughts and memory

Another big clue about depressed thinking is that you may feel as if your head is full of fog. Difficulty remembering even recent things or in concentrating on everyday tasks can get in the way of getting things done. At times like these, it can be hard going to make decisions or to work at your usual pace. Temporarily reducing your expectations of yourself and setting smaller achievable goals are among the strategies recommended for dealing with these changes.

DIFFERENT KINDS OF DEPRESSION

Many different clusters or combinations of depression symptoms are possible, including atypical, psychotic and mixed depression.

Atypical depression

The experience of depression may be subtly different for people with bipolar disorder and those who have unipolar depression (where only depression is experienced, not hypomania or mania). A pattern of so-called *atypical depression* may occur more often in people with bipolar disorder. One of the reasons this pattern is called atypical is that instead of having insomnia, loss of appetite, and being very sad and tearful, which are all characteristic of unipolar depression, people need to sleep and eat more, and feel flat and slowed down when depressed. You may feel temporarily better when good things happen, but this does not change your underlying mood. Marked fatigue and sensitivity to rejection are also common in atypical depression (Cuellar et al., 2005).

Psychotic depression

For some people with bipolar disorder, extreme negative thinking can take the form of psychotic delusions, including beliefs about excessive personal guilt, such as believing that you have committed a sin or a terrible crime, or paranoid delusions, such as believing the police are out to get you. Hallucinations are occasionally present. In psychotic depression, however, psychotic symptoms accompany the symptoms of depression. Psychotic depressions typically respond to medical treatment:

> I really believed that I was guilty of ruining my children's lives by being an inadequate parent and of causing the natural disasters that had recently hit the world. The way I was feeling (my depression) was God's way of punishing me for this. **George**

Mixed depression

You may have mixed depression if you have a major depressive episode (see chapter 1) plus some symptoms that are typical of hypomania or mania at the same time. The number of manic symptoms required for a depression to be considered a mixed state is not certain, but recent studies suggest that you need to have at least three hypomanic or manic symptoms (Benazzi, 2007). These often include irritability, racing thoughts, talkativeness, agitation or distractibility. It is important to know whether you have a mixed depression, because for some people, antidepressant medications may aggravate rather than reduce these moods. Tim discovered that he sometimes experienced a mixed depression:

> Everything was dark and I felt oversensitive. The usual friendly faces just irritated and annoyed me. Sleep did not come easily and I could not sit still and my thoughts raced but I felt tired and run down. Nothing gave me enjoyment. I was restless and just felt on edge and thought how worthless I was and how little point there was to anything.

HOW SEVERE IS YOUR DEPRESSION?

The experience of depression in bipolar disorder ranges from having only a few mild symptoms to having frequent or severe episodes. You may find it helpful to work out a list of symptoms that you typically experience in an episode of depression or/and mixed depression. A template for the list is available at www.eburypublishing.co.uk/bipolar. This can help to identify your typical warning or early symptoms, as explained in chapter 10, which means that you can implement strategies for managing your depression before it gets too severe. Recognising symptoms that may persist between episodes provides the opportunity to address and minimise these too.

A full episode of depression

The diagnosis of a full major depressive episode involves a cluster of five or more persistent symptoms (for at least two weeks), one of which is either depressed mood or loss of pleasure in things. Episodes range from mild to severe depending on how intense the symptoms are and how much they interfere with your daily life, relationships and safety. It is important to note that the symptoms of depression are not always static throughout an episode. For example, some people report a progression from lethargy and feeling flat, to severe negative thinking and suicidality as they start to gain more energy. The frequency and duration of a person's depressive episodes also vary.

While medical treatment is standard for depressive episodes, research has found that medication combined with psychotherapy may be most helpful in reducing depressive relapse in bipolar disorder (Scott & Colom, 2005). Appropriate support from others has also been found to help protect people from depressive relapse and to shorten the duration of depressions (Johnson et al., 1999). Personal strategies to manage symptoms of depression and prevent or reduce relapse are discussed in more detail in chapters 11, 12 and 17.

Mild depression lasting a few years

Some people with bipolar disorder experience a slightly milder ongoing version of depression (at least three symptoms) that has continued for two years or more. This is called *dysthymic disorder*. Tina, a teacher with bipolar II disorder, explains her experience of dysthymia:

> It was not like my usual severe episodes of depression when for a few weeks I would experience very severe darkness, when I stopped enjoying anything, hated myself and the world, couldn't get up to go to work and just wanted to sleep or to end it all. This cloud had been around for a few years now. It dulled my usually sharp memory and concentration, sapped my energy and my confidence, made it harder to go to work, or to make the effort to be sociable. I still managed to work and enjoyed playing the piano and walking on the beach with my pets, but I was not myself. It was as if I was waiting to regain that lively person who enjoyed life.

People sometimes don't recognise that they are living with a mild depression that may be interfering with their lives, and which may respond well to a combination of medical and psychological treatment and personal coping strategies.

A few symptoms between episodes

Some people are still left with a few symptoms of depression, which can hang around for months like an uninvited guest, even when the full depressive episode is over. These lingering symptoms are sometimes referred to as *residual* or *subsyndromal* symptoms; they might not be too bothersome and can clear up reasonably fast. But other times residual symptoms can disrupt everyday life and require treatment in their own right. Residual symptoms may make it harder to cope, and increase your risk of relapse (Perlis et al., 2006).

Paul, a 40-year-old man with bipolar disorder, related: 'It's six months since I left hospital after an episode of depression, and although my mood has improved and I can enjoy things again, the insomnia and lack of energy saps me. It's a real struggle to return to work.'

One theory about the symptoms of depression that linger between episodes is that in certain cases they may be misunderstood and ignored and considered to be part of a person's personality. Lingering depression can also be a result of the debris of illness. Recovering from episodes can be stressful as you wade through the backlog of accumulated tasks and demands and this may play a role in perpetuating depressed feelings. Take things slowly and set small manageable goals to get back on your feet. Sometimes the disruptive effects of bipolar disorder on your relationships, career and self-esteem may contribute to feeling depressed. It can take time to come to terms with the illness and the changes it brings and to create a fulfilling life with bipolar disorder.

Lingering symptoms may respond to medical treatment, lifestyle changes and psychotherapy, and people develop personal strategies that effectively reduce them. Sometimes, despite your best efforts, they can persist and seem to be part of your 'normal mood'. Although it is not easy, people manage to structure their lives to accommodate these lingering symptoms. If you experience this type of depression, it does not mean that you have failed to control your illness; it means that some forms of depression are more resistant than others.

Warning signs and early symptoms

For some people with bipolar disorder, depression happens abruptly, hitting them like a lightning bolt out of a clear sky, with no warning. Others notice early signs or symptoms of the depression developing. These are sometimes referred to as 'prodromes', as they may precede the full episode, and thereby act as a warning. For example, you may be much more sensitive to criticism than usual and believe that people are rejecting you, and you might start cancelling arrangements. Sometimes people only recognise that they are becoming ill when the episode begins. Although prodromes can be difficult to identify, getting to know the subtle changes in feeling, thinking and behaviour that are your early symptoms of depression can help you to take action and reduce the risk of relapse.

KEY POINTS

- Most people with bipolar disorder experience depression.
- Depression is not who you are. It involves changes in the way you feel, think and behave that are part of an illness.
- Depression is more intense, persistent and disruptive than the temporary lows everyone experiences in response to everyday ups and downs.
- Depression may at times feel devastating and overwhelming, but it is treatable.
- People can have different combinations of depressive symptoms; sometimes depressive symptoms may be combined with symptoms of hypomania or mania.

- You may experience different levels of severity of depression. Making a list of the symptoms that you typically experience as an episode of depression can assist you in identifying milder symptoms and those that may be warning signs of an impending episode.
- Some people have a few depressive symptoms between episodes; finding ways of managing these may make a difference to everyday life.
- Identifying your warning signs or early symptoms of depression is not always easy, but catching them early can mean recovering more quickly.

3 MANIA AND HYPOMANIA

Colours are bright and the light glistens. My thoughts dance from one idea to the next, quick, sharp and brilliant. Words tumble out my mouth. I keep moving and do not notice your concerned faces. **Tess**

Everyone with bipolar disorder experiences mania and/or hypomania at some time. Different levels of severity and different combinations of symptoms may render your experience a bit different to that of another person with the same illness. Hypomania is a milder form of mania. Symptoms of these elevated or 'high' mood states can range from extreme exuberance to a quieter, elevated confidence that is nonetheless marked by activity. Depending on your symptoms, the experience of hypomania or mania can be pleasurable or exhilarating, or unpleasant, confusing and very distressing. However, the pleasure or exhilaration often comes at a cost, due to the unfortunate consequences of symptomatic behaviour or the subsequent fall back into depression. This chapter examines more closely some of the changes in feeling, thinking and behaviour that occur when people are hypomanic and manic. You may recognise your own experience here.

HOW SEVERE IS YOUR MANIA/HYPOMANIA?

As with depression, mania and hypomania can involve a range of degrees of severity and different clusters of symptoms. It can be useful to develop a list of the typical symptoms you experience in an episode of hypomania or mania and the website connected to this book provides a table where you can list your symptoms. This can help you to develop a summary of the warning signs that you get before an episode develops so you can catch symptoms early and prevent relapse.

An episode of mania or hypomania

An episode of mania or hypomania involves either elevated, expansive or irritable mood plus a cluster of at least three symptoms (four if your mood is irritable), as noted in chapter 1. These symptoms may include increases in activity, risk taking, pleasure seeking, sex drive and speeding up of thoughts and speech, increased self-esteem, as well as a decreased need for sleep.

Mania

Certain things people do when manic, such as engaging in risky sexual activities or financial schemes, challenging people and buying things they can't afford, can have serious consequences. When mania becomes very severe, some people experience psychotic symptoms, such as delusions or hallucinations and marked changes in their thinking. Others do not experience psychosis, but the mania still gets in the way of their everyday lives. Many people with bipolar I disorder experience a period of hypomania on their way up to mania.

Hypomania

The distinction between mania and hypomania is one of severity. When hypomanic, people do not experience the same degree of disruption to their daily functioning, require hospitalisation or develop psychotic features as they may in full manic episodes. People with bipolar II disorder who experience hypomania but not full mania often feel more creative, better able to function at work and socially, and better able to achieve their goals when their mood is a little elevated. Lori Oliwenstein describes mild mania or hypomania in her book *Taming Bipolar Disorder*:

> When you are in an early or mild mania, or when you are hypo-manic, the world truly is your oyster. The energy feeding into you opens your mind just a little wider and gets you moving just a little faster. It lets you reach a little farther for what was previously just beyond your grasp (Oliwenstein, 2004:46).

The darker side

Hypomania is not always a wonderful experience, as it can often involve increasing irritability, over-sensitivity and feeling uptight and restless. This can affect important relationships. Likewise, many people experience 'dysphoric mania', in which some of the key manic symptoms are combined with some symptoms of depression. This can be a much more disturbing experience. In classical mania, you may feel euphoric, over-confident and excessively optimistic as part of your experience of mania. In mixed mania, besides having manic symptoms such as increased energy, decreased need for sleep, racing thoughts and speech, you may feel depressed, guilty, suicidal, fatigued, anxious, and irritable or agitated, and your mood can be labile (changeable). This experience can be distressing and there is an increased risk of self-harm, so immediate treatment is essential.

To diagnose mixed mania, DSM-IV requires full features of both a manic and depressive episode to be present, but some research suggests as few as two or more of the following depressive symptoms—depressed mood, loss of interest or pleasure in things, suicidal thoughts, guilt, fatigue or anxiety—mixed in with manic symptoms, may be sufficient for diagnosis (Cassidy et al., 2000).

Treating episodes

The most effective treatment for hypomanic and manic episodes is considered to be medical treatment. Ongoing use of mood-stabilising medications has shown excellent results in reducing the future risk of manic episodes, pointing to the strong biological causes of this mood disorder. Dealing with other factors that trigger an episode, or catching symptoms early, may also help prevent relapse.

A few symptoms

People with both bipolar I and II disorder occasionally find that they have a few symptoms left over from an episode of hypomania or mania. Some of these, such as sleep difficulties, can get in the way of daily functioning whereas others, such as an increase in goal-directed activity, might be less disabling. Because these mild symptoms can interfere with strategies for staying well, such as sticking to a regular sleep and activity routine, it is recommended that people seek treatment for them.

Warning symptoms

Warning symptoms or prodromes of hypomania and mania are not difficult to identify (Lam & Wong, 1997), providing you with the opportunity to nip the episode in the bud or reduce its severity and consequences. Studies show that identifying early changes can help you to reduce relapse and to function better at work and socially (Perry et al., 1999; Lam et al., 2001).

WHAT CHANGES WHEN YOU BECOME HYPOMANIC OR MANIC?

A number of changes in what you do, how you feel and the way you think occur when you become hypomanic or manic.

Activity changes

Look out for changes in your behaviour, as they are often the easiest changes to pick up. You or others may notice that you:

Do more than usual

This increase in activity may appear to be organised and productive, especially early on, and then become more frenetic and extreme. Sara notes: 'When I am becoming hypomanic I start cleaning the house and find it increasingly hard to stop for a break or to get some sleep.'

Restlessness and agitation
You may become restless and move from one task to another, or so agitated that it feels impossible to sit still, let alone achieve your goals.

Need much less sleep
You may feel that you have a lot of energy and don't need to sleep as much as usual. For many people, sleep difficulties and a reduction in the number of hours they sleep are telltale signs of growing hypomania or mania.

Become more talkative
Your speech may become faster, louder and more pressured, so it is harder for people to interrupt you or to have their say.

Try to achieve more goals
You may direct much more of your attention and time to pursuing your goals, often at the expense of your usual activity and sleep routine and other urgent responsibilities. Goals can become more numerous and unrealistic the more ill you become.

Forget to eat
Basic physical necessities like eating sometimes feel unimportant when becoming manic, and people seem to survive with little food.

Take more risks and act impulsively
Initially you may notice a slight change, in that you are significantly less cautious at work or drive a little faster, and are more eager to share your opinions in social situations. You may pursue pleasure more intently and become sexually more provocative in the way you dress, or spend money more freely.

For some people these subtle changes signal the onset of the more serious risky behaviour that occurs when manic, such as reckless driving, entering suspect business deals, making rash decisions including ending relationships, dangerous sexual encounters, and excessive use of alcohol or drugs, gambling and spending sprees.

Change the way you relate to people

When people are hypomanic, they often seem to know just the right things to say, are full of ideas and are engaging company, but they may also become irritable, snappy and defensive when contradicted or thwarted. As your mania increases, you can become intrusive, socially inappropriate, impatient, argumentative and paranoid. As Tom, a musician, reports: 'I phoned everyone I knew in the middle of the night, even distant acquaintances.'

Irritability and aggressiveness

People who are experiencing dysphoric mania may be very irritable or sometimes aggressive. Friends, family and workmates can often feel that they have to tiptoe around them in order not to spark off verbal or occasionally physically violent outbursts, which are some of the more severe symptoms of this phase of the illness.

Bizarre behaviour

This is part of psychotic mania, as demonstrated by Charlie, who ran down the road in his pyjamas, declaring that he was the Messiah.

Feeling manic or hypomanic

There are noticeable changes in how you feel as you become hypomanic or manic, with feelings becoming more intense. This may include:

Mood elevation or euphoria

You might notice that you feel much better than usual, to a degree that is unrelated or disproportional to what is going on in your life at the time. In its milder forms, mood elevation involves a pervasive sense of wellbeing, as if nothing can go wrong. In hypomania, there may be a milder, more channelled excitement. Mood elevation can increase to intense, irrational elation and excitement, regardless of realistic demands or problems.

Loads of energy
You may feel as if you can keep going for hours and need little rest.

Heightened senses
Hypomania and mania seem to enhance colours and natural beauty. Sounds, smells and tastes are magnified.

More spiritual or religious
People report mystical experiences of unity with nature or God.

Increased sex drive
Some people report an increase in their appetite for sex.

Increased self-confidence and self-importance
Some people have a greater sense of their own power, and feel able to achieve anything. They may feel that what they do, who they are, or what they have to say has some special significance or importance. When manic, people may feel bulletproof. Such moods impose a self-assurance that is evident to others. To the outsider, people in a hypomanic or manic state are very convincing. It is the difference from how they usually are, the gaps in logic, and their risky and strange behaviour, which alerts those close to them to their condition and creates worry and concern.

More sociable
Some people feel more of a need to relate to others.

Increased sensitivity
Some people can be defensive and sensitive to criticism of their ideas and schemes.

Irritability

Feeling irritable or angry in general, or specifically with others who cannot keep up with your pace or who censure your risky ventures, is not uncommon. Some people switch abruptly from euphoria to extreme irritability, and this makes it difficult for both you and others to know what to expect next. Anger can have unfortunate consequences if you act impulsively.

Impatience and impulsiveness

It may be difficult to wait or postpone being satisfied, or to give up wanting something even if it is risky or dangerous.

Being up but feeling down

Although you have many typical manic or hypomanic symptoms, you might feel sad, tired or anxious and have some symptoms of depression as well.

Spinning out of control

People sometimes feel as if they are losing control due to their impulsivity or psychotic symptoms. This can also be a very frightening experience for those who care about them.

Manic and hypomanic thinking

Changes in what you think of yourself, others and the future, and in the way you think are common, and include:

Seeing yourself as powerful

You may see yourself as powerful and able to do great things. In hypomania, such thinking may not be too unrealistic and extra confidence can even be helpful. As you become more ill, your view of yourself may become more grandiose and unrealistic. Some people make commitments to enormous and challenging or risky projects that they later regret.

Thinking becomes self-focused

As hypomania develops there is increasing absorption with your own needs and gratification.

Seeing the world through rose-coloured glasses

People overestimate luck and the helpfulness of the world. They can become blind to risk, and end up doing dangerous things that can have damaging effects on their life.

Viewing others in extreme ways

When you become hypomanic or manic, judgments about others range from very positive, overestimating their good qualities or attractiveness, to hypercritical. In the same way, you may consider that other people have extreme positive or negative views about you.

Thinking more negatively

If you experience mixed mania, your thinking may actually have more in common with the pessimism and negative thinking about yourself and others that is common to depression.

> I felt a sense of dread about the future. I moved from one task to another trying to get things done but my thoughts raced and I kept thinking of something else I needed to do. My mind was awake with thoughts about all the terrible things I had done in the past and I could not sleep. My partner's concern irritated me. Instead I drove very fast to a nearby casino and decided to see if I could beat fate and win some money. **Jim**

Racing thoughts

When you are mildly hypomanic, thoughts may seem quick, but as you become more manic they seem to run away with you.

Muddled thinking

When you are hypomanic, your thinking may seem to be to the point and clear, but this can change, with your attention wandering from one irrelevant detail to the next. If this mood state intensifies, you might become so distracted that it is hard to concentrate on one train of thought or to remember things. In the extreme forms of mania, people jump from one series of ideas to another based on only the loosest of connections. For example, while you are talking about a shopping expedition your thoughts may suddenly jump to the Apollo expedition on the moon. To the observer, when these thoughts are expressed in speech they do not make sense. Seeing unusual connections between things, combined with creative energy, has led to great artistic works and ideas from people suffering from bipolar disorder. However, muddled thinking can squash some of this creativity.

Loads more ideas

People have lots more ideas and plans when becoming manic, which often results in productive action, but as mania gets worse their ideas can become more unrealistic and bizarre. Chasing after numerous goals can disrupt sleep and usual routines, increasing your spiral into mania.

Increasing belief in your ideas and opinions

As people become more manic, they often become more convinced of the value of their ideas. There is also often an increasing sense of urgency to act on these ideas.

Bizarre thinking

Some people develop delusions (fixed beliefs that have no basis in reality) about their special talents and authority or, in more dysphoric mania, paranoid delusions about how people are against them. People can have auditory and visual hallucinations in which they hear and see things that are not really there, or ideas of refer-ence when they think they are receiving special messages. John reports: 'I believed the newsreader on TV was telling me to stand for president and I had to immediately start my election campaign.'

THE BURDEN AND THE BEAUTY

Some people with bipolar disorder may miss hypomania and even 'euphoric' mania. The temporary wonder, productivity and sense of success sometimes linked with these mood states may seduce people to prolong their hypomania or mania rather to take steps to treat it. Occasionally, people even seek it out by doing things that may trigger mania, such as stopping treatment or taking stimulants. Unfortunately, they are often left with the disruptive consequences of euphoric mania. The other problem with such elevated moods is that they seldom stay positive. Many people slide into the distress of depression or mixed mania. For most people who experience hypomania and not mania, it is the frequency or seriousness of their depression that makes them decide to seek treatment:

> Rita, a 27-year-old marketing assistant, explained that when she was hypomanic she got so many wonderful ideas and had so much energy to put them into practice. A few weeks later she would crash, and sit at her desk doing nothing and wishing she could be in bed. It was as if she had burnt herself out. She discussed this problem with her GP, who explained that she had typical symptoms of bipolar II illness, and she began treatment.

Remember that mania is not your fault. The things you do when manic are part of the illness. The pain of shame and guilt following a manic episode, and the strain on family relationships, can bring additional stress in the recovery period and contribute to depression. As a result most people actively seek treatment and strive to bring their bipolar disorder as much under control as possible and to make the most of their life.

KEY POINTS

- All people with bipolar disorder have episodes of hypomania and/or mania at some stage, which may vary in severity and in terms of the combination of symptoms experienced.
- Becoming familiar with your pattern of hypomania or mania can help you to reduce the impact of bipolar disorder on your

life and help your loved ones to understand your illness and be supportive.

- Making short lists of the typical symptoms you experience in a hypomanic or manic episode, and your warning signs, can help you to monitor your illness and take action to prevent or reduce episodes when necessary.
- Disturbing and disruptive behaviour is a symptom of illness and not your fault.
- For some people, the experience of hypomania or mania involves pleasure and productivity, but this is short lived and soon transforms into depression or mixed states.
- Even when mania is a pleasant experience, it can have devastating consequences on relationships, occupations and financial security.
- Effective treatment involves medication, psychotherapy and personal strategies, which are explained fully in later chapters.

4 ADAPTING TO BIPOLAR DISORDER

*Which of the me's is me? The wild, impulsive, chaotic, ener-
getic, and crazy one? Or the shy, withdrawn, desperate,
suicidal, doomed, and tired one? Probably a bit of both, hope-
fully much that is neither.*

Kay Jamison, *An Unquiet Mind*, 1997:68.

Living with bipolar disorder involves not only the symptoms, but
also how the illness affects your life. It is a very personal experience, and many people find it hard to come to terms with. In this
chapter we look at different approaches that people take to adapt
to life with bipolar disorder, ranging from denying that you have
the illness to attributing everything to it, or actively pursuing the
elevated moods. Somewhere between these extremes is another
approach, which involves a basic acceptance of the disorder and
flexible movement between a focus on illness and a focus on life,
depending on the severity of your current symptoms. Some
people move between the various approaches at different points in
their life; many find a way of managing that helps them to control
their illness as much as possible and lead a full life.

DENIAL WHEN FIRST DIAGNOSED

Consider what it was like for you receiving the diagnosis of bipolar disorder. Sometimes there is an element of relief when you are diagnosed. Jake, a 25-year-old whose extreme mood swings got in the way of his final years of school and his relationships, explains: 'It took 10 years to get the right diagnosis but at last my moods are being treated and I am able to get on with living my life.'

Receiving this diagnosis can lead you to ask yourself deep questions about who you are and what it means in terms of your future. The image you have of bipolar disorder when you are first diagnosed may be influenced by misconceptions and stigma about mental illness. It is not surprising that some people react with defiance and attribute their symptoms to external causes, such as work stress, diet, exhaustion and conflicts, or to their personality.

There are also milder forms of denial. 'Under-identification' may involve some acknowledgment of the disorder, but without real acceptance or ownership (Miklowitz, 2002). This kind of denial can mean knowing that you have bipolar disorder but wanting to forget about it, and not properly following through with treatment or lifestyle changes. This reaction is common in other illnesses as well. For example, people with heart conditions may acknowledge their diagnosis but put thoughts about it out of their mind, neither stopping smoking nor changing their diet. Ultimately, a certain amount of acceptance is necessary in order to manage your illness, but this can take time. The experience of having more than one episode increases the realisation that the illness needs to be accommodated.

> For many, the first step to wellness is to be given the correct diagnosis. The next step is to accept the diagnosis. When people accept their illness, and learn about it, they are often able to take more control of their lives (Russell, 2005:127).

Dealing with painful emotions

Denial can be a way of protecting yourself from some of the more painful emotions that can arise as you come to terms with your bipolar disorder, such as anger, fear, shame, guilt and sadness. These reactions may reappear from time to time as you find ways of living with your illness.

Some people with bipolar disorder have described a grief process whereby they mourn for the healthy person they thought they were, and the losses and changes resulting from their illness. If you have experienced sadness when faced with such loss or change, you are not alone. Chris explains how concerned he felt about his relationship after his first episode of mania:

> After the episode, I knew things had changed between us. I cannot describe the sadness and the fear. I wondered if she could again see me as the person she had known and trusted for so long. It would take time for us both to take in what had happened and to recover our relationship.

Managing your bipolar disorder can involve finding new ways of seeing yourself that both recognise your strengths and talents and take into account your vulnerability to the illness. It can also mean coming to terms with the losses, and developing new sources of meaning and fulfilment.

Shame and humiliation

Some people experience shame and humiliation when learning about their diagnosis. You may feel like this when you have recovered from an episode in which you did things that do not sit well with your standards and who you are. There are times when it can be important to remember that 'bipolar disorder is something that you have, but it is not who you are' (Miklowitz, 2002:56).

You may blame yourself rather than the illness for the understandable drop in status that sometimes results from being ill and for not being able to live up to certain expectations and standards.

Bipolar disorder can affect your attention, memory and daily functioning and some people become distressed and despondent when they cannot live up to the standards they have set for themselves in life. Periods of illness may make it difficult to achieve what you set out to do and the stress and pressure involved in chasing unrealistic goals may make you more vulnerable to relapse. Some people with bipolar disorder tend to set particularly high standards and push themselves to achieve unrealistic goals (Johnson 2005, Lam et al., 2003). Recovering your self-esteem may involve considering your strengths, abilities and what you enjoy and finding alternative manageable and meaningful goals, which take the limitations of the illness into account.

Stigma about the illness and its consequences can make shame and humiliation worse. It can be particularly hard to see beyond the stigma if those close to you share it. Denial can be a way that both you and your loved ones deal with this stigmatised illness. As Francis said: 'We just ignored my growing depression and everyone was polite while my world was crumbling and I could not work and withdrew for days to the seclusion of my bed.' A problem with denial is that it delays or prevents effective treatment.

Even people who have lived with bipolar disorder for a long time can find that the experience of stigma remains demoralising. A vital part of dealing with stigma is to see through the misconceptions it involves and to hold on to who you are besides the illness. Reports from people who live with mental illness show that it is possible to accept that you have bipolar disorder and still feel good about yourself, assert your rights when necessary and lead a full life (Young & Ensing, 1999).

Guilt

Some people feel guilty about having bipolar disorder, as if they have somehow brought it on themselves. While people can do their best to control their bipolar disorder, it is still a biological illness. Having bipolar disorder is no more your fault than having asthma is the sufferer's fault. Guilt and shame may also arise from the consequences of behaviour when ill, as is evident from the American poet Robert Lowell's words:

> I want to apologise for plaguing you with so many telephone calls last November and December. When the 'enthusiasm' is coming on me it is accompanied by a feverish reaching to my friends. After it's over I wince and wither (Goodwin & Jamison, 1990:19).

It can be vital when well again to be able to see that it was your illness at work, even if you have to face the consequences of these actions.

Anger

As with other chronic illnesses, it is natural to ask: Why do I have this? Why me? At times you can feel very angry about the illness and the limitations and losses, and family members may feel the brunt of your anger. Sometimes it can be useful to find some constructive expression for this anger, such as painting or writing. The anger often dissipates when your illness is effectively treated, and you begin to feel more confident and enjoy life again. Still, it is only human to feel angry or frustrated from time to time when confronted by something that appears so unfair.

Fear

In the beginning there is so much that is not known: what bipolar disorder really is, and what it means about you and your future. This can either result in fear and efforts to avoid thinking about the diagnosis or in constant worry and efforts to prevent relapse. Finding out more about bipolar disorder and effective ways to control your illness and make the most of life can help to reduce this fear.

What helps?

After a few episodes of illness, the reality of the disorder and the effectiveness of ongoing treatment often lead people to find a bit more peace with their diagnosis, as they discover that they can manage their bipolar disorder. Louise, who has been living with bipolar disorder for a long time, once said that it took a number of episodes before she gave up denying that she had it:

> It irritated me that people kept trying to remind me about my illness. In the end, I realised that each time I stopped treatment I got sick again. It just wasn't worth it. Now having been on treatment consistently for the past two years, I have experienced fewer episodes, and my floristry business is going well.

Discovering that you have bipolar disorder can be a confusing time, and it may be helpful to discuss these feelings with a trusted clinician, to get more information about different kinds of bipolar disorder and treatment possibilities, and to speak to people with bipolar disorder who have found ways to reduce episodes as much as possible and enjoy life. There are some helpful books written by people with bipolar disorder and international peer support organisations listed on this book's website.

DENIAL AFTER MANY EPISODES

Coming to terms with bipolar disorder is not always an all or nothing phenomenon, however. Even after many years, denial may still be a way of avoiding frustration with the limitations imposed by your illness, the disruption of a few ongoing depressive symptoms, or the disappointment or trauma of relapse. Sometimes, even after many episodes, denial is a way of protecting yourself from the hurt of stigma.

Bipolar moods can make people question their diagnosis. Depression can feel very true to life sometimes, leading people to believe that this is how things really are and they are not ill at all. Rejection of the illness and the need for treatment more commonly occurs when people become manic, however, regardless of how many episodes they have experienced. These practical difficulties sometimes require making plans when you are well, with your clinician or others, about how you wish to manage these phases if they arise.

Being well for a long time may encourage people to underplay or question their diagnosis and the need for treatment. Sometimes people who have had bipolar disorder for a long time feel the need to test whether it really is a recurrent illness or even whether they were correctly diagnosed, so they stop their medications or do not maintain their regular sleep cycle. Such testing is understandable, but can put them at real risk.

BECOMING YOUR ILLNESS

Some people who accept the diagnosis of bipolar disorder go to the opposite extreme to denial, and see themselves 'as' the disorder. The positive side of this approach is that you do acknowledge your illness, and a focus on illness can be useful when you are developing symptoms, as it can help you to get well. Seeing yourself as the illness is understandable if you are currently ill or have experienced many episodes or have rapid cycling. The negative side is that severely cutting yourself off from life when you are well may be denying you the chance to rebuild and enjoy your life.

Over-acceptance of or 'over-identification' with your illness can mean that everything that happens, even when you are well, is explained by the bipolar disorder (Miklowitz, 2002). For example, if you are feeling well but have an argument with a colleague who has been rude, you may automatically blame your reaction on your illness rather than the rudeness.

While people with bipolar disorder may have the hard task of adjusting to certain changes in lifestyle and necessary limitations, they sometimes place excessive and unnecessary limitations on themselves and their lives. This may occur if they feel very anxious about relapsing. Angela, who has been well for the last two years, explains: 'I do not want to socialise or to get involved in things as I have to take it easy because of my bipolar disorder. I do nothing and feel frustrated and unfulfilled, but I can't risk becoming ill again.'

An approach to illness that does not include a focus on living well, within the limitations imposed by the illness, can be very disempowering and make you feel unnecessarily hopeless and despondant. However, it is not always easy to see the difference between necessary and unnecessary limits—in other words, the balance between controlling your illness and enriching your life is not always easy to find. Through experience, you may learn to give both sides of the scale enough weight to make the most of your situation and stay well, as Jill, who has lived with bipolar disorder for 15 years, explains:

It takes time to figure out what works for you. When I am well, I still take my medications regularly, keep one eye on my moods, and watch for stressors, such as family arguments, or when my grandmother died last year. My other eye is on my life, everyday things, and the things I still want to do and my husband and kids. I approach things differently. For example, there was a course I wanted to do to upgrade my skills, and I had to work out a way to do it that would not be too stressful. I have learnt the times when I need to start being more vigilant of my illness and the times when I keep my bipolar there, but at the back of my mind.

SEEKING SYMPTOMS

Seeking out stimulants or other means of becoming hypomanic or manic, as some people do, comes at a cost. Living with uncontrolled mania, mixed states or the darkness of depression, and the resulting havoc in your life and the lives of loved ones, is a big price to pay. The alternative may be trying to gain as much control over your symptoms as possible, so that you have a chance of experiencing enjoyment, creativity and success when well without having to deal with the consequences of untreated illness.

LIVING WELL

The process of coming to terms with your illness has been called 'recovery', described as 'a deeply personal, unique process of changing one's attitudes, values, feelings, goals, skills and/or roles. It is a way of living a satisfying, hopeful, and contributing life even with limitations caused by illness' (Anthony, 1993:15).

This term has been criticised, however, as it gives the impression that recovery is some endpoint, a finite holy grail. When talking about an illness that involves recurrent episodes and, for some people, the experience of mild symptoms between episodes, recovery may be an ongoing process that is easier at some points than at others. We think that coming to terms with your illness may be conceptualised as a journey, a lifestyle or way of living with bipolar disorder that involves learning through trial and error what works for you in managing your illness and making the most of life.

The 'journey' approach is about an active acceptance and coping that involves taking control of things. It involves taking into account your bipolar disorder and your environment at a particular point in time and using appropriate strategies to try to maintain wellness. The way you manage your illness will change depending on the phase of illness—for example, you may need to focus your attention on preventing relapse or getting better while in hospital, or on taking things slowly rather than rushing to complete accumulated tasks after an episode of illness. When you are well, besides attending to any ongoing symptoms, and using strategies to keep well, you may be freed up to focus more on the rest of your life.

Your personal qualities, abilities and values

Appreciating your personal qualities can make it easier to live beyond stigmatised labels, and to make the most of your life. It can also help others to see and relate to the person behind the illness, and to know when you are becoming ill. Bipolar disorder can make you feel a bit fragmented and cut off from yourself at times. It can be difficult to experience a consistent sense of who you are when, for example, you may be gregarious and manic at one point and shy and withdrawn at another. People sometimes lose touch with their strengths and talents and what they value in life when they have been ill for a while. It can be easy to confuse your symptoms with who you really are, and other people can fall into the same trap. Perhaps one of the most important forms of stigma is self-stigma.

Self-stigma

Self-stigma comes about when you believe the stigmatised labels attached to being a 'mental patient'. You consider that this is who you are rather than viewing yourself as a person and your bipolar disorder as an illness. In doing this you are accepting the opinions of people who do not understand that there is more to you than your illness. The same thing happens when people believe any kind of prejudice against them—for example, that they are inferior in certain ways because they belong to a certain religion or have a certain skin colour. Self-stigma can deeply affect your sense of self-worth and limit your confidence so that you cease to recognise or express your qualities and strengths. Living according to a label constricts your identity. Of course, there are restrictions placed on you by your illness, such as, perhaps, needing not to overdo the socialising in order to stay well, even when you are a very sociable person, but self-stigma increases the restrictions. Coming to terms with your bipolar disorder can mean overcoming your own prejudices about mental illness, and affirming your unique identity.

Understanding the biological nature of bipolar illness and rebuilding yourself and your life may help combat the effects of stigma from within. David explains:

> I find it helpful to remind myself that having a disabling and debilitating illness that requires specific treatment and puts limitations on my life does not mean that I am less worthy than others. Like everyone else, I am a person with different qualities, strengths and vulnerabilities.

Getting to know yourself

Doing things that you enjoy, or that give you a sense of being in harmony with your beliefs, values, talents and strengths, can provide a sense of fulfilment when your mood is stable or even if you have a few symptoms of depression. Getting to know yourself, your illness and what is possible in your circumstances can assist with this.

It is not always easy to identify your abilities and positive personal qualities, and some people can be more familiar with their faults and limitations. It is better to consider this when you are well, as both being elevated or depressed can distort your perspective. When considering your abilities, think of numerous possible skills such as those connected to your work, hobbies, sports, interests, relationships and daily life. Some common strengths are listed on www.eburypublishing.co.uk/bipolar, and you can see which may apply to you.

It may feel like you were a different person before your bipolar disorder. Although the illness sometimes temporarily hides peoples' qualities and abilities and restricts what they can do, it can also lead to discovering new talents or interests or using old ones in new ways.

The following questions may help you with this discovery and some people also find it useful to get some input from someone who knows them well.

- What abilities, talents or positive personal qualities have I noticed in myself over the years?
- What skills do I enjoy using when I am well?
- What aspects of myself would I appreciate in a friend?
- What things have I enjoyed doing?
- What has interested me previously? (Areas to look at include work, hobbies, socialising and different kinds of activities like cooking, woodwork, cycling and art.)
- What values do I believe in? (E.g. helping others; people or animal rights; spiritual or religious beliefs?)
- Are there new skills or interests that I would like to develop, and how can I arrange this?
- What things are possible for me to do within my current situation (see SMART goals, chapter 18)?

Rebuilding

Rebuilding yourself and your life may require taking into account the realistic restrictions imposed on you by your illness and creating a good life for yourself within these limitations. You will then be in a good position to set realistic goals and participate in life in a way that is rewarding and reaffirming (see chapter 18).

> Jerry, a chef by profession, was having a hard time getting his episodes under control and found the demands of late nights at the restaurant very stressful. He took time off work and decided to stay at home and cook wonderful meals for his family when he felt up to it. As his illness got more under control, he resigned from the restaurant and slowly built up a successful part-time catering business preparing meals for people who were too busy to cook for their families.

Bipolar disorder affects everyone differently. Some people with bipolar disorder manage to continue in the same occupation while coping with their illness, others find different ways of expressing themselves and enjoying life. Usually, however, people make some lifestyle changes to adapt to getting the most out of life and keeping well (see chapter 18).

Dealing with external stigma

People with bipolar disorder are confronted at times with misconceptions, prejudice and discrimination. More appropriate education needs to replace misconceptions and fear. Nevertheless, attitudes to mental illness are changing due to successful treatment, advocacy and legislation. The availability of effective treatment is arguably the greatest influence in reducing stigma. Legal resources also give people more choices about standing up for their rights.

Many people report that expressing who they are through their participation in life gives them a better perspective on their illness, and the confidence to make choices if their rights are infringed. The consumer advocacy groups mentioned on the website associated with this book can help with information about your rights and legal resources.

To disclose or not?

Linked to stigma is the question of whether or not to disclose your illness to other people. The feeling of not being accepted or respected can be a painful experience, and lead to avoiding situations in which your illness may be revealed. Some people mix with others with bipolar disorder to avoid stigma. Others tell a few trusted people. Some people disclose their illness only to the human resources department at work or to their boss. Still others have come 'out of the closet' and declared their illness to the world. Public figures such as Professor Kay Jamison of Johns Hopkins University and Associate Professor Neil Cole of the Monash Medical School, who have talked openly about living with bipolar disorder, may have helped to reduce some of the misconceptions about mental illness. Disclosure is a personal decision, and you need to look at the pros and cons of disclosure in your particular situation.

As more accurate information replaces misconceptions in the public arena, such choices may be easier. If you have weighed up the situation, perhaps spoken to other people in similar situations, and have decided to disclose your illness to someone, there may still be a few things to consider. Conveying your view of yourself as more than just your illness, and of your illness as manageable, may encourage other people's confidence in you and enhance understanding of your bipolar disorder. How much information you provide may depend on what you think the other person needs to know. In certain situations you may decide not to use the term 'bipolar disorder' when explaining your illness, perhaps disclosing that you have 'a medical problem related to my energy level that can affect my work and concentration' (Miklowitz, 2002:282).

In other situations it may be appropriate to use the term 'bipolar disorder' and to give more detailed information. To help those who are close to you to understand your bipolar disorder, it is useful to use language and examples that the person you are addressing will relate to and easily understand.

Depending on the circumstances, you could include all or some of the following information:

- An easily understood definition of bipolar disorder.
- The fact that it is a medical illness.
- Effective treatments are available, which means that you may have isolated episodes that can be controlled, and may or may not be mildly symptomatic between episodes.
- Between episodes, you may be the same as the person they know you to be. Your behaviour changes significantly only when you become symptomatic.
- An explanation of how your work or relationship may be temporarily affected when you are ill.
- Ways in which another person may respond if they notice symptoms of illness.

KEY POINTS

- People find different ways of adapting to their bipolar disorder between the extremes of rejecting it and deliberately seeking it out. They may live through their illness and unnecessarily limit their engagement with the outside world when well, or seek out the highs and increase the unfortunate consequences of depressive or manic episodes.
- Denial of your bipolar disorder can be a natural reaction, especially when first diagnosed, and at times later on. When denial prevents you from constructively managing your illness, it becomes problematic.
- It can take time to come to terms with your bipolar disorder, and some people go through a grief process, which may reoccur to some extent at different times.
- Adapting to your bipolar disorder can mean accepting your illness and the need for ongoing treatment and strategies, while simultaneously carving out a life and identity for yourself within the restraints imposed by your illness. This is part of an ongoing journey that involves adapting to the different phases of your illness and making the most of daily life.
- Knowing your personal qualities, abilities and values can help you to see through the stigma attached to mental illness and to stand up for your rights.
- You can decide whether you would like to disclose your illness or not, and how much information to give in specific circumstances.

5 CAUSES AND TRIGGERS

The good news is that although you can't control your biology and, therefore, can't control having bipolar disorder, you can control the course of the disorder itself through medication, psychotherapy, and being aware of the environmental factors that play into your disorder.

Lori Oliwenstein, *Taming Bipolar Disorder*, 2004:62.

One of the questions that trouble many people who have bipolar disorder is why the illness happens. What causes bipolar disorder? Some people may answer 'family arguments' or 'work stress' and, indeed, different kinds of stress may trigger the illness—but stress is not the underlying cause. The underlying cause, as with any other illness, is biological. You can influence the course of your bipolar disorder by using constructive strategies to prevent or reduce relapse.

STRESS VULNERABILITY MODEL

Biological vulnerability refers to a person's predisposition to experience the symptoms of a particular illness. This vulnerability is present even when you are not experiencing symptoms. People can have biological predispositions to all kinds of illnesses, such as asthma, hypertension and diabetes. In the case of bipolar disorder, more is known about the factors that trigger relapses and influence the course of the illness than about the factors that spark off the first episode (Johnson, 2005); though we do know that abuse in childhood is a risk factor that may trigger bipolar disorder, though it is certainly not the only thing.

Factors that are known to trigger biological vulnerability are often lumped together under the heading of 'stress'. Stress is a pressure or demand placed upon us that comes from the environment (for example, family conflict) or from ourselves (for example, high expectations). A certain amount of stress may provide just enough of a challenge to have a motivating effect on a particular person's life, whereas too much stress for that person can be a burden that affects their health. It is as if certain stressors wake up the dormant biological vulnerability and result in symptoms. These stressors do not have the same effect in people who do not have a predisposition to bipolar disorder. Typical stressors that can trigger bipolar episodes include:

- major stressful events or accumulation of daily problems
- overstimulation
- disruption to sleep or activity levels
- chasing your goals
- interpersonal conflict
- drugs and alcohol
- physical illness
- stopping helpful medication.

The presence of a stressor does *not* automatically mean that it will trigger a bipolar episode, but it may increase your risk if you are vulnerable to that particular stressor. You will be more sensitive to stressors if you are already a little symptomatic. The advantage of being able to identify your personal triggers of illness is that you can take steps to minimise their influence on your mood.

Sometimes episodes of illness occur without any trigger. You may find that you become more sensitive to stress with more relapses, so that it takes less stress to spark you off than before. Some people find that as they have more episodes, mood swings occur more often even without any obvious major stressor to spark them off.

The stress vulnerability model includes the view that if biological factors such as genetics are strong—say, because there are several people in your family who have had bipolar disorder— you may need only a slight stressor to spark off the illness (such as a few late nights). People have individual stress thresholds (Miklowitz, 2002). Not all stressors will affect people with bipolar disorder equally, and it can be useful to work out those that set off your symptoms in order to find ways to reduce their hold over your life.

You have an important role to play, in that despite biological vulnerability and stressors, the way you cope and manage your illness can influence whether or not you will relapse. For example, drowning your sorrows in alcohol may make you feel more depressed in the long run whereas making sure your sleep is not disrupted when you are trying to meet work deadlines may help prevent hypomania. When you notice the presence of triggers, focusing attention on dealing with them can make a difference in preventing relapse. Managing your triggers, together with taking medications, having psychotherapy, following a healthy lifestyle, and responding to warning symptoms in order to prevent relapse can help reduce the impact of bipolar disorder on your life.

BIOLOGICAL VULNERABILITY

Biological vulnerability to bipolar disorder includes genetic factors, changes in the brain, including changes in brain chemicals, structure and functions, as well as hormonal and immune changes in the body.

Genetics

Bipolar disorder tends to run in families but it is not entirely a genetic disorder. Children of a parent with bipolar disorder are seven to twenty times more likely to have bipolar disorder than children of parents who do not have bipolar disorder. Yet that fact alone does not prove a genetic cause.

Identical twins share all their genes. In twin studies, identical twins are compared with non-identical twins who, like other brothers or sisters, share about half of their genes. When one identical twin has bipolar disorder, the other has a 60 to 80 per cent chance of also having it. In siblings or non-identical twins, the risk is only about 20 per cent (Smoller & Finn, 2003). If the disorder was 100 per cent genetic, all the identical twins would develop the disorder. Since this is not the case, while genetics may be a contributing factor, other factors must also be involved.

Multiple genes rather than a single gene are thought to be involved in bipolar disorder, which makes it harder to pass it on. Indeed, bipolar disorder is found in only 10 per cent of children who have a parent with bipolar disorder (Kelsoe & Niculescu, 2002).

People with bipolar disorder often worry about passing the illness on to their offspring, but remember that this is not certain. Either way, if you have children you will have an advantage in knowing about bipolar disorder and its treatment should one of them develop the illness. These days bipolar disorder can be detected early, and effective treatment may do away with much of the suffering that late diagnosis and misdiagnosis has inflicted on people in the past.

A few factors complicate the genetic studies in bipolar disorder. Major (unipolar) depression is commonly seen in relatives of people with bipolar disorder. Depression, and possibly schizophrenia, are more common than bipolar disorder in relatives of people with bipolar disorder, and can similarly be caused by environmental as well as genetic factors. Family members of people with bipolar disorder are also more likely to use drugs and alcohol (Potash & DePaulo, 2000). Although some individuals who have a family history of bipolar disorder do develop a psychiatric illness, most never develop any psychiatric problems at all. The risk of developing bipolar disorder seems to be a combination of particular genes and particular environmental stressors.

This idea that a genetic vulnerability can interact with an environmental trigger is similar to our understanding of many other medical conditions. For example, if you have inherited a vulnerability to high cholesterol or high blood pressure, environmental factors such as poor diet, lack of physical activity, smoking and stress all contribute to your risk of developing heart disease. The treatment in this example is to take medication to lower your cholesterol or blood pressure and to make changes to your lifestyle (for example, stopping smoking, increasing exercise, improving your diet, reducing stress). This is very similar to managing bipolar disorder, where we use mood stabilisers to treat the underlying disorder and use changes in lifestyle (for example, reducing stress, developing good sleep habits, avoiding drugs and alcohol) and psychotherapy to reduce the risk of relapse.

Changes in the brain

Differences in the brains of people with bipolar disorder have provided valuable clues about the biological causes of this illness.

Brain chemicals

Bipolar disorder is caused in large part by chemical imbalances in the brain. Medications for the illness target these imbalances.

Neurotransmitters are the chemical signals that nerve cells in the brain use to signal each other, like chemical emails. One cell sends many different neurotransmitters to another in order to communicate. These include serotonin, noradrenaline, dopamine and gamma-aminobutyric acid (GABA). These chemical signals may be altered in amount or in the way they function in people who have bipolar disorder. Neurotransmitters are involved in regulating the limbic system, the area in the brain that controls mood.

Dopamine plays a key role in drive, reward and motivation. In mania, these moods are enhanced, while they are decreased in depression. A role for dopamine in causing bipolar disorder is also suggested by the fact that drugs of abuse such as amphetamines, which drive dopamine, can characteristically precipitate bipolar episodes.

The neurotransmitters bind to nerve cells at receptors, which behave like plugs and sockets. Once the neurotransmitters have connected with the nerve cells, other chemicals, called second messengers, are activated. There are a variety of second messengers, including proteins called G proteins, protein kinase C and calcium. These messenger systems are changed in people with bipolar disorder, and mood stabilisers such as lithium work on regulating second messengers (Brunello & Tascedda, 2003).

Nerve growth factors

The brain produces nerve growth factors, or neurotrophic factors, which are vital for the survival and functioning of particular nerve cells in the brain. A new theory suggests that a loss of nerve cells in some brain regions and a decrease in survival-promoting factors may be involved in bipolar disorder. Mood stabilisers increase nerve growth factors and can prevent some of the changes seen on brain scans of people with bipolar disorder (Bachmann et al., 2005; Chang et al., 2005). Early, consistent and appropriate treatment may prevent brain changes and improve symptoms and everyday functioning.

Clocks and sleep

If you're bipolar, you probably have an exquisitely sensitive body clock, one that responds quickly and almost violently to changes in the signals it receives (Oliwenstein, 2004:138).

Everyone has an internal clock that sets the body's many cycles, such as the sleep/wake cycle, which determines when you usually fall asleep and wake up. The body clock regulates the release of hormones and chemicals affecting vital biological functions, such as blood pressure, temperature and hormone secretion, which vary during the day–night cycle. The 'clock' is a tiny group of nerves called the suprachiasmatic nucleus, which is found in the hypothalamus in the middle of the brain. Genetics may have a role in setting an individual's body clock. People with bipolar disorder may have changes in the setting of the clock's speed, and lithium may affect genes that regulate this clock (Yin et al., 2006).

The factors that help set your body clock include regular activities, social stimulation and regular sleep patterns. The hormone melatonin is released in response to light, which is influenced by when you go to sleep and wake up, and helps control your sleep/wake cycles. People with bipolar disorder are particularly sensitive to changes in daily rhythms such as sleep and activity patterns. Jet lag and shift work, major life events such as a death in the family or moving house, or more minor changes such as changing working hours, may cause disruption to your daily rhythms and affect your body clock. Even a single night of sleep loss can trigger mania in a sensitive individual. Sleep loss can both cause mania or hypomania and become a symptom of illness, increasing the severity of the mania (Leibenluft & Suppes, 1999).

Some people with mood disorders have been found to have more episodes of depression when the reduction of light in autumn, and particularly in winter, affects melatonin. About 20 to 30 per cent of people with bipolar disorder have this vulnerability, with hypomania or mania peaking in spring when daylight hours increase (Hallam et al., 2006).

Immune changes

The immune system is the body's defence against infection. It uses both immune cells and chemicals to fight infection. There are subtle changes in immunity in people suffering from both ordinary depression and bipolar disorder (Wadee et al., 2002).

Hormones

Cortisol is a hormone secreted by the adrenal glands at times of stress. There may be excess cortisol in people with bipolar disorder (Thakore & Dinan, 1996). Cortisol has effects on the brain, and excess cortisol may affect nerve cells. New medications aiming to treat bipolar disorder by working on cortisol are under development.

KEY POINTS

- Biological causes of bipolar disorder include genetic predisposition, changes in the brain (including brain chemicals, structure and activity in some brain regions), changes in the regulation of the body clock, as well as immune and hormonal changes in the body.
- Rather than a single pathway to illness, an interaction between biology as an underlying vulnerability, and a variety of stressors as triggers, may result in an episode of illness for a particular individual.
- You can influence the course of your illness and prevent or reduce relapse by using constructive coping skills such as medications combined with psychotherapy, managing your triggers and warning symptoms, and leading a healthy lifestyle. Similarly, destructive ways of coping, such as using alcohol or drugs, can make your illness worse.

6 MEDICATION AS A PERSONAL STRATEGY

Although staying well is rarely just about taking prescribed medication, medication is an important component of many stay well plans. To be more precise, the right medication at the right dose . . . even when feeling good.

Sarah Russell, *A Lifelong Journey*, 2005:129.

Medication has proven to be an effective first-line treatment for bipolar disorder and is recommended by sufferers themselves. Despite the usefulness of medication, about half of the people who are prescribed medication to treat their bipolar disorder stop taking it or do not take it regularly or at recommended doses. There are many reasons for this, ranging from side effects to sometimes mistaken beliefs about bipolar disorder and its treatment. Using medication as a strategy to help you manage your illness is a personal decision. There is a lot at stake here, because stopping medication increases your chances of relapse, being hospitalised and the risk of suicide. In chapter 5, Causes and Triggers, we saw how medications act directly on biological imbalances. Not taking medication leaves you vulnerable to untreated illness.

This does not mean that you must stay on an unhelpful medication or one that is giving you unbearable side effects. Some people respond well to a particular medication; others may need to try different medications or different doses before finding what suits them. Giving medication a fair trial means taking it regularly, monitoring how it is affecting you, and being able to discuss things openly with your doctor so that together you can make the right treatment decisions.

In this chapter we look at some ideas for getting the most benefit from your medication and discuss frequently asked questions about using medication.

MAKING THE MOST OF MEDICATION

There are a number of things you can do to get the most benefit from your medical treatment:

- **Take medications regularly and reliably.** Taking prescribed medication regularly and reliably will give it a good chance to work, and you can find out whether taking a certain dosage at a particular time of day is or is not helpful. Taking medication as it is prescribed also enables the right level to build up in your body.

- **Get information on your medications and see how they are affecting you.** Knowing the potential benefits and side effects of your medications, and how long they take to work, can help you to assess if a particular medication is working for you. You can monitor how the medication is affecting you, the positive effects on your mood and on preventing relapse, and side effects (see chapter 16), and use this information when making treatment decisions with your doctor. Your previous experience about what works and what does not is valuable in guiding treatment.

- **Communicate with your doctor.** Developing a good relationship with your doctor, so that you can talk openly about your doubts or concerns, can make it easier to sort out medication problems. You can ask your doctor for information and treatment options. Your doctor needs to know about your symptoms, how the medications are affecting you, and if you are on other medications or have any other health problems besides bipolar disorder. Regular doctors' appointments and blood tests (when necessary) can help you to keep an eye on how things are going. If you are becoming ill again you can contact your doctor to discuss your medications. Some people have medication that is prescribed in advance by their doctors so they can adjust their intake medication if they are becoming ill. Scheduling extra appointments if you notice warning signs or symptoms can be helpful, as you and your doctor can monitor things together and work as a team in trying to prevent or reduce relapse.

- **When considering stopping a medication it can be helpful to:**
  - discuss your concerns with your doctor, and weigh up the pros and cons of stopping a medication as Tony does in table 6.1;

Table 6.1 Tony's pros and cons

Pros (List the benefits and advantages of taking medications.)	Cons (List the disadvantages and difficulties of taking medications.)
Mood more stable and don't need to go to hospital as often, can finish what I start, less reckless spending and embarrassing sexual affairs so good for my relationship, can consider return to work	Hands shake, dry mouth, always having to remember to take pills and get scripts and blood tests, reminds me that I have bipolar disorder

- think very carefully about stopping or changing something that is working for you, unless you have unbearable side effects. Remember that taking the right medication at the right dose can prevent and reduce relapse, reduce your risk of hospitalisation and suicide, and protect you from some of the negative consequences connected to bipolar episodes;
- check with your doctor to see whether you need to gradually stop the medication;
- postpone decisions about stopping medication if you are becoming ill again.

FREQUENTLY ASKED QUESTIONS

Using medication for bipolar disorder is not as simple as taking antibiotics to clear up an infection. Many people have questions about using medications (Miklowitz, 2002; Basco, 2006). These include:

Can I stop my medications as I am well now?

Medication can help to prevent or reduce episodes while it is in your system, but once it is out of your system the protection wears off. For example, you may feel fine initially when you stop lithium, but the chances of relapsing within a few months are very high. Relapse will occur even more rapidly if this medication is stopped *abruptly* rather than *gradually*. Ongoing treatment with lithium has been shown to reduce suicide attempts and completed suicides (Tondo & Baldessarini, 2000).

A mood stabiliser such as lithium will not work if you take it only when you feel ill, because the medication needs to reach optimal levels in your blood. Stopping and starting medication or taking it erratically can mean that it takes longer to reach these levels. Then you may be judging its effectiveness when it has not had a good chance to work. You could discuss these matters with your doctor before making a decision.

Is my medication addictive?

There is no evidence that any of the medicines widely used in bipolar disorder are addictive. This is different from the fact that people can relapse when stopping mood stabilisers, as relapse occurs because the bipolar disorder is untreated. Benzodiazepines such as diazepam can be addictive, but these are not part of long-term management for most people.

I miss my elevated moods. Can I take less medication and keep the highs?

For some people hypomania and euphoric mania can be positive or pleasurable experiences, and they do not want to treat them. The reality is that hypomania and euphoric mania come at a price. Mania has disruptive consequences. If you choose to live with these moods, you are very likely to experience the other side as well: the depressions, dysphoric manias and/or depressed mixed states. Taking mood-stabilising medications can help to reduce not only your highs but also your depressions and other disruptive mood states and their consequences.

After living with bipolar disorder for a long time and weighing up the costs and benefits of pursuing her seductive hypomanias, Kay Jamison concluded: 'I am too frightened that I will again become morbidly depressed or virulently manic—either of which would, in turn, rip apart every aspect of my life, relationships, and work that I find most meaningful' (Jamison, 1997:212).

There is no evidence that taking your mood stabiliser in less than prescribed amounts will result in a 'slightly manic' rather than a fully manic state.

Will I be too stable or blunted when taking medication?

Some people complain that they are too stable or blunted when taking medication. It is a matter of weighing up the pros and cons of stability for you personally. 'Stability puts you in the driver's seat and gives you more control over your fate than the illusion of control that mania gives you' (Miklowitz, 2002:135).

Stability does not have to mean that your feelings are blunted. Although the feeling of being blunted could result from your particular medication, it could also be connected to your being accustomed to experiencing more extreme feelings. After years on the roller-coaster, intensity of feeling becomes 'normal' for some people, and losing that exhilaration can seem strange. It can take time to become used to life without the mood swings. Some people find that stability offers them the ability to feel alive and be creative again. Jerome, for example, said:

> My passion is composing music and before my bipolar disorder was diagnosed I had pages of music, unfinished sheets lying all over the house. I am using a number of strategies including taking medication and making sure I get enough sleep to calm my moods. Since my illness is more under control I have completed pieces of music and have got a contract to compose, so I will be able to earn money from my passion.

If blunting is a side effect of your medication, it is sometimes possible, in consultation with your doctor to fine-tune your medication so you are less blunted and your mood remains stable.

Is medication a sign of weakness, a need for a crutch? Is it controlling me?

Some people see taking medication as a sign that they cannot cope without a crutch. To these people, being in control means not relying on anything else. Being independent is a good feeling, but even very independent and capable people make use of resources to achieve their goals. Taking medication can be a way of taking control and using the available resources to achieve your goal of staying well.

We are all vulnerable to the biological side of our beings. When we are hungry, we need to eat, for example. It is important not to forget that although bipolar disorder is a personal experience, you still have an underlying biological vulnerability. The fact that there is no physical evidence of illness does not mean that bipolar disorder requires no medication.

Taking control of your illness by using the strategies available for managing it can give you more control over your life. Making the most of medication requires that you control your medication and actively monitor and assess its effects in order to decide on the best treatment. Your medication strategy may help to stabilise your mood and put you in the driver's seat.

What can I do about side effects?

As can happen with medications for all sorts of different illnesses, the medications prescribed for bipolar disorder may involve side effects. People often comment that some doctors just don't know what it is like to have to put up with side effects. It can be very helpful for you to discuss openly with your doctor how a medication is affecting you, and what the side effects mean to you. Your doctor may be able to suggest alternatives, such as possible dosage changes, taking the medication at a different time, alternative or additional medications, or tips for managing some of the side effects.

How can I remember all these instructions about taking my medications?

Starting a new medication is sometimes like trying to remember a new language. What may help is to try to develop a medication routine, so that taking the medication becomes like brushing your teeth, as does recording its effectiveness and side effects. Some people find that it helps to connect medication times with other aspects of their routine, such as mealtimes or feeding the cat, which they do at the same time each day.

If you take many different medicines at different times, your pharmacist can package them into a Webster pack, which is a pack with all your tablets packaged together in blisters, labelled to tell you when to take them. Using a dosette (or pillbox) and placing it somewhere that will remind you to take your medication can be helpful.

It sometimes helps to schedule regular doctors' appointments in advance, as well as blood tests, so you know they are in your diary. If you run out of medication, try telephoning your doctor for a repeat script that will last until your next appointment.

How can I afford the medication?

The high costs of medication can be very difficult. If you are routinely finding that your income just isn't stretching far enough, seeing a financial counsellor can help you look at your budget with new eyes and work out how things could be improved. In an emergency, welfare agencies often provide emergency relief funds for essentials such as medication.

Is it dangerous to take medication?

Some people are scared of taking medication and of certain side effects and long term treatment. Check whether the side effects you are concerned about are actually possible with that medication, and discuss your worries with your doctor. If medication is properly taken and monitored by you, with regular blood tests if necessary, and regular visits to your doctor, the rare risks can be well controlled. It is also useful to see the risks of treatment in balance against the risks of untreated bipolar disorder.

What can I do if I can't find the right medication?

It is common for a particular medication to work for one person but not another, and for people to respond better to certain medications than others in different phases of the illness. Combinations of medicines can be useful when a single medication is not fully effective. Your medications may need to be adjusted to suit the different phases of your illness.

Sometimes it is hard to find a medication that works for you. You may build up hopes and expectations around a new medication, only to have them smashed when it does not work. Feelings of disappointment and frustration are normal. Remember that there are many options, such as changing the dose or the medication and adding other medications. Your doctor will be able to provide more information on your options. It is useful to have a doctor or confidant who you can talk to and who will encourage you to persevere in this trial and error process of finding the best medication regime for you.

Should I continue my usual medications if warning symptoms appear?

Despite maintaining your ongoing strategies to keep well, warning signs and early symptoms sometimes appear. These may be a signal to consult your doctor to assess whether you need to adjust your medication to help prevent or reduce relapse. Some people have a prearranged agreement, based on experience, about taking additional medication when they find they are becoming hypomanic or manic or are unable to sleep.

What does taking medication for bipolar disorder say about me?

It can be hard to see beyond the stereotyped and stigmatised image of mental illness. Sometimes people refuse to take medication because they believe doing so confirms they have a mental illness. Similarly, relatives or friends may actively discourage taking medication as a way of denying your illness. Remember, you are more than your bipolar disorder, and it is important to see through this stigma in order to take action and reduce the hold bipolar disorder has over your life.

What taking medication may really be saying about you is that you have the guts to take control, to confront the options and take responsibility for creating a good life for yourself. Facing any recurrent illness can lead people to make decisions and to live life more consciously than they might have done, and this may be particularly true of bipolar disorder. You may need to take a stand and follow what you know is right for you.

KEY POINTS

- It is clear that using medication helps many people to gain more control over their bipolar disorder and thus allows them to enjoy the other aspects of their life. Although medications can be so effective, about half the people with bipolar disorder do not use them in ways that enable them to reap these benefits.
- There are things you can do to make the most of taking medication and to play an active role in your treatment.
- People have many questions about taking medications, and you might find that some of the comments in response to common questions in this chapter stimulate more discussion between you and your doctor over related issues or concerns that are important to you.
- Far from the idea of medications controlling you, making the most of this potentially life-changing strategy means taking control of your medications to manage your bipolar illness.
- Taking medications can be included as a central strategy together with your other strategies for managing your bipolar disorder. There is more information on medications for bipolar disorder in the next chapter.

7 GETTING TO KNOW YOUR MEDICATIONS

Finding out more about my medications and monitoring how they affect me has helped me to take charge and make sensible treatment decisions with my doctor. **Andrew**

The discovery half a century ago that lithium can both treat and prevent relapse in bipolar disorder revolutionised our understanding of the illness, and the lives of many sufferers. Bipolar disorder can now be managed over the long term with appropriate treatment so people can potentially live regular lives. This may eventually contribute to its destigmatisation. In the last decade, many new treatments have been introduced, and an unprecedented number of novel treatments, both medication and psychotherapy, are now under development. This should further increase hope for people with the disorder and their families.

For some people, taking the medications that are right for them can almost completely remove mood swings; for others, good medical treatment may both reduce the severity of their mood swings and make them occur less often. It is still possible, however, to experience 'breakthrough episodes' while on medication so that your doctor may need to alter the dose or include another medication.

Knowing about medications can assist you in getting the most from your medical treatment and reducing the impact of bipolar disorder on your life. This chapter provides some introductory information about medical treatment. First, we discuss how medications can help in the different phases of illness, then we take a closer look at mood stabilisers, atypical antipsychotics and other medical treatments.

All medications have two (sometimes more) names. One is a generic name which reflects its chemistry, the other is a brand name given by the pharmaceutical company producing the medication commercially. Because brand names vary from country to country, in this book we use the generic names.

MEDICATION AND PHASE OF ILLNESS

Medication is used differently in the different phases of the disorder, and is often targeted to specific symptoms.

Mania and hypomania

A number of medications are effective in the treatment of mania and hypomania alike. Lithium can treat manic and hypomanic episodes, either alone or at times in combination with other medication. The advantage of lithium is that the same treatment for the acute episode can remain the cornerstone of long-term treatment. Lithium is most predictably useful if you experience hypomania or mania with elevated or euphoric mood (classic mania), and where there is a family history of bipolar disorder. Other useful treatments include medicines initially used to treat epilepsy, such as valproate, also known as divalproex, and carbamazepine. Atypical antipsychotics, which include olanzapine, risperidone, aripiprazole, clozapine, ziprasidione and quetiapine, are all clearly effective for the treatment of mania, both alone and in combination with other mood stabilisers.

When mania is mild, the use of a single medicine may be sufficient. If mania is more severe, or you have an episode when you are already on appropriate treatment, it is often necessary to add a second mood stabiliser.

The choice of medication is based on a number of issues. Overall, these medicines are equally effective. However, there are factors that guide choice, including how well a medicine has worked before, how well it has agreed with you in terms of side effects, whether you have other illnesses, its financial cost to you, and whether it has been useful in treating your family members. Medicines differ subtly in that they may be more effective in treating certain kinds of mood. As an example, lithium is more useful in mania that is euphoric, and valproate and atypical antipsychotics in mixed mania. People can respond to a medication in many individual ways, and there is unfortunately no easy way to predict a response. Ultimately, this means that the choice of medication and finding what works for you needs to be based on experience and discussion between you and your doctor.

Depression

The treatment of depression in bipolar disorder is complicated. Antidepressants on their own are not recommended, as they can cause hypomania or mania, mixed phases and rapid cycling. The treatment of depression in bipolar disorder involves taking a mood stabiliser if you are not already on one, or optimising your present mood stabiliser treatment, and possibly adding a second one. If you are still depressed, an antidepressant may be added. Antidepressants may be combined with mood stabilisers if you have severe or persistent depressive symptoms, a long-term illness pattern of severe depressive symptoms with few hypomanic or manic symptoms, or severe suicidal impulses that have not responded well to mood stabilisers alone. All antidepressants must be used for a few weeks before they take effect.

Authorities are divided as to how long to continue antidepressants once they have worked, with most believing that mood stabilisers should be the foundation of long-term treatment. While there is minimal evidence that antidepressants used over the long term prevent bipolar relapse, nevertheless a few people may benefit from long-term antidepressant treatment. The atypical antipsychotics, including quetiapine and olanzapine, and mood stabilisers, particularly lamotrigine, are also used to treat depression.

Mixed states

In a mixed state, depressed symptoms may be more obvious than manic symptoms, and people are often misdiagnosed as having depression. This can be problematic, as mixed states respond best to the typical treatments for mania rather than to treatments for depression. The key to the treatment of mixed states is the recognition that the types of treatment that are useful are similar to those that are useful in mania, namely mood stabilisers and atypical antipsychotics. Antidepressants are not useful in mixed states, even when your symptoms are predominantly depressive or you are feeling suicidal, as they can make your mixed state worse.

Recognising mixed states early and accurately is essential, as the best treatment is quite specific and takes time to be effective. A combination of medicines may be necessary to treat mixed states. Additional mood stabilisers often need to be used to settle a mixed state. Atypical antipsychotics such as olanzapine are also helpful in the treatment of mixed states.

People tend to take longer to recover from mixed states than from manic or depressed episodes. You need to take this into account when you assess whether a treatment is helping you or not. A very common issue is for people to feel that treatment is not working, when either they or their clinician is persuaded to stop treatment or make changes too quickly. Stopping a mood stabiliser can make mixed-state symptoms worse. Therefore, it is important to be patient with mood stabiliser treatment of a mixed state and not to bail out before the medication has had time to work, which can take several months.

Rapid cycling

Knowing that you have rapid cycling bipolar disorder is valuable information, as its treatment is different from that of non-rapid cycling illness. For many sufferers of rapid cycling, the dominant mood, or the one that causes the most distress in the cycle, is depression, which often fails to respond to what seems to be adequate or appropriate treatment. As in mixed episodes, rapid cycling can be aggravated by antidepressants, and mood stabilisers are beneficial. Lithium has clear value in the treatment of rapid cycling, although the response is not as robust as in non-rapid cycling patterns. Valproate, lamotrigine and atypical anti-psychotics may also be useful. Rapid cycling often needs multiple mood stabilisers for adequate control. Rapid cycling, like mixed states, can take many months to settle. If you are taking appropriate mood stabilisers for rapid cycling, it is important to persist with them long enough to allow them to take effect.

Maintenance treatment

Most people with bipolar disorder want not only to reduce an episode of illness when it occurs, but also to prevent relapse. With recurrent episodes, new episodes tend to come more frequently. Conversely, the longer you are well, the longer you are likely to remain well. The key to controlling your illness is therefore the prevention, as much as possible, of new episodes. Due to the biological risk of developing an episode of bipolar disorder, relapse is always a possibility, and medication is usually seen as a long-term treatment.

A mood stabiliser is used for maintenance treatment, which is ongoing treatment to prevent new episodes of depression, mania or mixed states. Lithium is still generally regarded as the gold-standard maintenance treatment. Other maintenance treatments include valproate, carbamazepine, lamotrigine and atypical antipsychotics such as quetiapine, olanzapine and aripiprazole. You may find one medication more helpful than another, as each has different clinical properties and potential side effects. It is also common to need more than one maintenance medication, as it is possible to have only a partial response to a single medication.

Treatment of anxiety

Some people with bipolar disorder have prominent anxiety symptoms that need to be addressed along with their bipolar symptoms. If you have high levels of anxiety you are more likely to be prescribed benzodiazepines, although how helpful they are in the long term is not entirely certain. It is important to recognise that benzodiazepines are addictive, a quality which can cause other problems, and to discuss this with your doctor. While antidepressants are frequently used in anxiety disorders for people who do not have bipolar disorder, in bipolar disorder there are concerns that they can trigger rapid cycling and mixed states. There is no evidence that antidepressants help anxiety in the context of bipolar disorder, and mood stabilisers remain the foundation treatment. As the underlying mood state resolves, anxiety tends to dissipate. Atypical antipsychotic medications (see section later in this chapter) have anti-anxiety effects, and psychotherapy is important in augmenting medical treatment to reduce anxiety in people with bipolar disorder.

MOOD STABILISERS

A 'mood stabiliser' is defined as a medication that is effective in stabilising manic, mixed and depressive episodes and/or in preventing new episodes from developing if taken regularly in an ongoing way. A medication can be defined as a mood stabiliser only if it does not contribute to rapid cycling or bring about the opposite mood episode. For example, a medicine you take when depressed should not increase the risk of having a manic or hypomanic episode. Mood stabilisers help you to regulate your mood swings but do not take away their cause, thus you need to keep taking them in order to prevent relapse, rather than taking them only when you have an episode of illness. They can be used in combination with other drugs or on their own. We discuss the most commonly used mood stabilisers: lithium, valproate, carbamazepine and lamotrigine.

At this stage, how mood stabilisers work is not fully understood. They have effects on cell signalling, altering the passage of information between nerve cells. They alter some neurotransmitters: lithium affects serotonin, valproate works on GABA, atypical antipsychotics block dopamine, and lamotrigine has an impact on glutamate. Some have effects on sodium and calcium channels in cell membranes. Lithium also seems to affect the body clock that regulates biological rhythms. Most mood stabilisers increase nerve growth factors, the proteins that have a role in promoting the survival and growth of neurons. Many have antioxidant properties. Mood stabilisers can also prevent the subtle brain changes sometimes seen in bipolar disorder.

Lithium

Lithium is the oldest and best-established treatment for bipolar disorder. It is given as lithium carbonate, a naturally occurring salt. Although initially used to treat active mania, it is now also used as a maintenance treatment to prevent new episodes. It also has an important role in both the treatment and the prevention of depression. It has value in rapid cycling and mixed states, but it is especially useful in people who have classical mania or hypomania.

There is good evidence that lithium can help you to control bipolar disorder, and abruptly stopping it can be a powerful trigger for a new episode. Going on and off lithium may make it less likely to work the next time you take it. Most importantly, the incidence of suicide and serious suicide attempts is substantially reduced during maintenance lithium treatment. Lithium may be compared to insulin, used to control diabetes. Insulin does not cure the disease, but it helps to control symptoms so that the person with diabetes can lead a more normal life. If the insulin is stopped, symptoms of diabetes reappear.

Lithium is seldom effective immediately. It can take weeks or months before you notice an improvement, and further improvement may gradually occur as you continue to use it. It is important to give lithium time to work.

Most people can use lithium, but if you have heart, kidney or thyroid problems, discuss these conditions with your prescribing doctor before taking it. If the dose or blood level of lithium is too low, it will be ineffective, and if it is too high, side effects can develop. It is essential to monitor levels of lithium with regular blood tests, which allows you to get the maximum benefit from the medication and minimise risks. It is also necessary to monitor body functions that can be affected by lithium treatment. Lithium can sometimes lower thyroid function and very occasionally affect kidney function (Schou 1977). As lithium is excreted in urine, the efficiency of your kidneys affects the medication's blood levels.

Lithium levels can become too high if the dose you are taking is too high, or you become dehydrated from vomiting and diarrhoea when ill, from heavy sweating in hot weather or from exercising or using hot baths or saunas. Some medications, such as diuretics (water tablets), anti-inflammatory and some blood pressure medicines can also push up lithium levels. It is essential that you do not start any new medicine without checking with your doctor or pharmacist that it is compatible with your lithium treatment. If your lithium levels become too high, you may experience lithium toxicity. The signs include persistent diarrhoea, vomiting or severe nausea; trembling, weakness or twitching of hands or legs, blurred vision or slurred speech; unsteady gait or dizziness, or swelling of feet and lower legs. If you experience any of these signs, contact your doctor immediately as lithium toxicity can be dangerous.

Remember the importance of checking your lithium levels, because when they are in the correct range there is a greater chance of the medication being effective. It is also necessary to take lithium precisely as prescribed. It is hazardous, for example, to double the dose if you forget a previous dose. The optimal dose of maintenance lithium needs to be decided by you through balancing, in collaboration with your doctor, three things: its effectiveness in reducing symptoms; optimum blood levels and any side effects. As changes occur in your mood, the dose may need to be altered accordingly. Regular appointments with your doctor are helpful in getting the most benefit from this medication.

Side effects

Side effects of lithium tend to be related to blood levels. The majority of people do not get most of the side effects listed below, although some people may have a few, especially when they are just starting out on lithium therapy: increased thirst, increased urination, nausea, mild stomach cramps, mental dulling, fine tremor of hands, mild sleepiness, slight muscular weakness, decreased sexual ability or interest, slight dizziness, occasional loose stools, weight gain, metallic taste, dry mouth and worsening of acne or psoriasis.

These side effects usually disappear or decrease after a few weeks of treatment. The most likely to persist are increased thirst, frequent urination, weight gain and fine tremor of the hands. It is important to discuss side effects with your doctor so that you can find the best possible dose with the least possible side effects. You might have a few tricks to deal with the side effects you experience. Some practical ideas that might be helpful in dealing with common side effects are listed in table 7.1. Because many of these are related to blood level, one option is lowering the dose, something which you would need to discuss with your doctor. A balance must be struck between keeping the dose low enough to be free of major side effects and high enough to be useful.

Pregnancy and breast feeding

Women who take lithium during the first three months of pregnancy may be at increased risk of giving birth to babies with certain heart abnormalities. Although the risk is very low, it is important to discuss these risks with your doctor, preferably before deciding to become pregnant. It is possible to plan gradual discontinuation of lithium and alternative treatment for these few months. The risk of a new episode needs to be balanced against the possible risks in pregnancy; it is also a risk to the baby for its mother to be ill. It is wise to discuss these issues with your doctor before conception. Lithium is excreted in breast milk. Breastfeeding has clear benefits to the baby, and here the risks and benefits of taking lithium need to be discussed with your doctor.

Valproate

Valproate, also available as divalproex, was initially used in the treatment of epilepsy, and a mood-stabilising effect was noticed in people using it. Like lithium, it is useful to treat mania and hypomania, and as an ongoing treatment to prevent relapse, and is sometimes used for depression as well. It may work a bit more quickly than lithium in acute manic states; also, it may be easier for you and your doctor to raise your dose more quickly without

Table 7.1 Managing side effects of lithium

Side effect	Helpful tip
Increased thirst and urination	Drink lots of water or suck ice cubes. Talk to your doctor about taking most of your tablets at night time or, if severe, trying a decreased dose may need to be discussed.
Persistent hand tremor	Taking lithium with meals or in frequent smaller doses may help. Cut down on caffeine (coffee, tea, cola drinks, chocolate), as caffeine may make it worse. If tremor is a severe problem, dose changes can be discussed. Adding another medication such as a beta-blocker may help. Switching to a slow-release lithium preparation is sometimes helpful.
Persistent nausea	Taking lithium with meals, taking smaller doses more frequently, or switching to a slow-release lithium preparation may be helpful.
Metallic taste	Take tablets with milk or water and food.
Skin rash, itching	This may be a sign of an allergic reaction to lithium or another possible cause, and you should consult your doctor.
Excessive weight gain	Try to begin a regular exercise program from the outset, even if it is only once or twice a week to start with; if you want you could build it up slowly. Exercise is important, as it is also beneficial for your mood. Another suggestion is to consult a

continued

dietician or weight reduction clinic to help
you make healthy eating habits a part of
your lifestyle (losing weight gradually and
maintaining it), rather than following a
strict diet, which you cannot sustain. Such
goals could be part of your plan to
maintain your wellbeing. *Note*: drastic
diets or fluid restriction should be avoided
since both can increase the risk of lithium
toxicity. Avoid diet pills with stimulant
properties since they may set off
depressive or manic episodes. Remember
to avoid high-calorie drinks.

significant side effects. If mood swings still occur, they are usually
less intense and less frequent. As with other mood stabilisers, it
may take many months before the full benefits of valproate are
achieved.

To get the maximum benefit from taking this medication,
monitoring of your medication routine, backed up by the
required blood tests and consultation with your doctor, is
necessary. Blood levels are less critical with valproate than with
lithium. Your doctor may also recommend a blood test for liver
functions and blood platelets, as very rarely this medication can
affect liver enzymes and production of blood platelets.

Side effects

Not all people taking valproate experience the possible side effects,
but you might find that you have one or two, like weight gain, which
is relatively common. Particularly at the start of treatment, you may
feel nauseous, sleepy or sedated, be a little unsteady on your feet, or
have indigestion or a hand tremor. It may be useful to take tablets

with water and after food. Slow-release tablets may cause less nausea, but can slightly increase diarrhoea. If side effects are severe, your doctor may suggest other medications to help reduce them, or check your blood levels and reduce the dose, or change the formulation of your pills and time schedule associated with taking them (for example, take more at night if valproate makes you sleepy). Less common side effects include swelling, visual changes and hair loss or thinning, which is usually transient and may be counteracted by zinc and selenium supplements. This medication can interact with other medications, including lamotrigine and carbamazepine, and it is important to consult your doctor or pharmacist before taking any other medication while on valproate.

Pregnancy and breast feeding

Valproate can cause congenital abnormalities in infants born to mothers who were on the treatment in the first months of pregnancy. The most significant of these is spina bifida, in which the spinal cord is open to the skin. Because of this, valproate is generally not used where pregnancy is a possibility.

Carbamazepine

Like valproate, carbamazepine was initially used as a treatment for epilepsy. In bipolar disorder, carbamazepine is useful to reduce acute mania or hypomania, and as an ongoing maintenance treatment to prevent relapse. It may work well for people who have not responded well to lithium, especially for those with mixed episodes, rapid cycling or psychotic manias. About a third of people who have not responded well to lithium will respond to carbamazepine.

As with the other major mood stabilisers, your doctor may start you on a low dose and raise it to maximise the advantages and reduce the side effects. Carbamazepine does not have a specific blood level that is clearly associated with the best response. Like the other mood stabilisers, carbamazepine needs to be taken regularly for months before its full potential to prevent episodes will be realised.

Carbamazepine can cause the liver to break down other medicines more quickly. This may make it necessary for your doctor to alter the dose of other medicines you are using, or to monitor them more carefully. Carbamazepine can reduce the efficacy of the oral conceptive pill. Because of the possibility of interaction, it is important to discuss all the medications you are on with your doctor before taking carbamazepine.

Certain tests can ensure the safety of this potentially effective treatment. In rare cases, carbamazepine can cause a serious drop in the white blood cell count, so your doctor may monitor your blood count regularly while on this medication. If you develop a fever, infection, sore throat, sores in your mouth, or easy bruising or bleeding, let your doctor know. People taking carbamazepine, slightly more often than on valproate, can develop a mild elevation in their liver enzymes and may need regular liver function tests. Sodium levels can also be affected, and kidney function may need to be tested. Thyroid levels need to be checked too, as, rarely, carbamazepine has an effect on the thyroid gland.

Side effects

Like all medicines, in a few individuals carbamazepine can cause side effects. Nausea, vomiting, constipation or diarrhoea can occur, but tend to improve with time. If your side effects are severe and persistent, you may need to discuss dose reduction, or splitting the dose over the day. Mild memory impairment (such as difficulty finding words) can occur. This is usually related to the dose you take, and is likely to disappear after several weeks or months of treatment.

Other side effects include blurred or double vision, drowsiness, unsteadiness or unusual tiredness. These tend to settle with time, but may need a reduction in dose. If you are feeling unusually tired on this medication, it may be useful to discuss checking your thyroid hormone levels with your doctor. Very rarely an acute allergic reaction can occur—if it does, you need to contact your doctor immediately. Signs of allergy include a severe rash, shortness of breath or swelling of the face. About 10 to 15 per cent of people report skin rashes, which also should be reported to your doctor immediately, as they can signal the onset of a more serious skin condition that may require treatment.

Lamotrigine

Lamotrigine is used in the treatment of bipolar depression and rapid cycling, but is less effective for mania. Lamotrigine is also used as an ongoing treatment, where it seems to be more effective in preventing depression than mania or hypomania. Most other mood stabilisers, including lithium, valproate and the atypical antipsychotics, may be better for preventing mania and hypomania than depression, but have some positive effects on all these mood states. Lamotrigine has been used to treat people who haven't responded well to other medications, either by itself or in combination with another mood stabiliser.

It arguably has fewer side effects than the other mood stabilisers. The most worrisome side effect is rash, which occasionally can be serious. To minimise the risk of rash, the dose must be increased very slowly. Being on valproate at the same time increases the risk of rash, so the dose has to be increased even more slowly. Other side effects tend to be relatively mild and usually transient, including problems with physical coordination, dizziness, drowsiness, nausea, vomiting and headaches.

ATYPICAL ANTIPSYCHOTICS

This group of medications is increasingly used for bipolar disorder. They include olanzapine, aripiprazole, risperidone, quetiapine, amisulpiride, ziprasidone and clozapine, medicines which were first used in the treatment of schizophrenia. Despite their name, their use in bipolar disorder has little to do with their effect on psychotic symptoms, and they all have independent effects on mood. Atypical antipsychotics can reduce mania and can be used alone or in combination with other mood stabilisers. Some of them also work for depression, especially quetiapine and olanzapine. Olanzapine and quetiapine prevent further episodes of illness, and are now regarded as mood stabilisers. Aripiprazole also has relapse prevention properties. Atypical antipsychotics can also relieve anxiety, restlessness and problems with sleep.

These powerful effects on your mood need to be weighed up against the side effects that are experienced by some people, which include sedation, tremor and blurred vision, dry mouth and loss of libido. In some cases these medications can increase cholesterol and glucose levels and aggravate diabetes, so you may need to monitor these factors with your doctor. Some antipsychotics cause movement symptoms including tremor, muscular stiffness and restlessness. Side effects can be minimised by using the lowest doses necessary for them to work effectively.

Different atypical antipsychotics have slightly different side effects. It is possible, together with your doctor, to choose the one that suits you best. For example, olanzapine and clozapine cause the greatest weight gain, while risperidone can cause more of the movement side effects. Clozapine is unique, having the most serious side effects, including being toxic to bone marrow and possibly to the heart, and requires the most intensive monitoring. Nevertheless, it may be a particularly useful reserve option for people in whom other medicines have been unsuccessful.

COMBINATION THERAPY

People with bipolar disorder often need combination therapy for effective mood stabilisation, because a single medication tends to reduce some but not all symptoms. Combinations of different mood stabilisers are increasingly used, and many people—perhaps the majority—will need to take more than one medication in order to become and remain well.

OTHER MEDICAL TREATMENTS
Antidepressants
It is not recommended to take antidepressants alone for treating bipolar disorder, as they can trigger hypomania, mania, mixed states and rapid cycling. In people who do not experience mania or hypomania and suffer from depression only (unipolar depression), antidepressant treatment on its own is beneficial.

The most commonly used antidepressants are the *selective serotonin reuptake inhibitors* (SSRIs): fluoxetine, paroxetine, sertraline, fluvoxamine, citalopram and escitalopram. These newer antidepressants tend to have fewer side effects than the older ones, and some help reduce anxiety as well. They have a somewhat lower risk of causing mania, mixed states and rapid cycling. Side effects can include nausea or diarrhoea when beginning treatment, and sexual dysfunction.

Dual reuptake inhibitors work on both serotonin and noradrenaline (also known as norepinephrine) and include venlafaxine and duloxetine. The dual reuptake inhibitors may also have fewer side effects than the older medicines, although the risk of triggering hypomania and mania may be higher than with the SSRIs. *Buproprion* is also an effective antidepressant in bipolar disorder.

Monoamine oxidase inhibitors (MAOIs) include phenelzine and tranylcypromine. MAOIs remain useful antidepressants, especially when newer treatments have not been sufficiently effective. They nevertheless are seldom prescribed as a first line of treatment, as they can cause a hypertensive crisis in which blood pressure is raised to dangerously high levels. It is necessary to be on a special diet, avoiding cheese and certain other foods which can interact with MAOIs and cause a hypertensive crisis. Side effects of MAOIs include low blood pressure, dizziness, feeling faint, dry mouth, fine tremor, constipation, blurred vision, reduced sexual response, indigestion, drowsiness and weight gain. If you have diabetes, epilepsy or any liver, kidney, heart or thyroid condition, or if you are pregnant, let your doctor know, as these drugs may have to be used with caution or avoided.

Tricyclic antidepressants are older medicines, and include imipramine, amitriptyline, desipramine, dothiepin and clomipramine. These, like the dual reuptake inhibitors, have a greater risk of inducing mania, as well as mixed states and rapid cycling, and are not often used unless other treatments have been unsuccessful. Side effects include dry mouth, constipation, blurred vision, weight gain, drowsiness and dizziness or fainting. If you have prostate problems, heart disease, epilepsy, hyperthyroidism, glaucoma, or are pregnant, tell your doctor, as this group of medicines must be used with caution in these situations.

Benzodiazepines

The benzodiazepines, such as clonazepam, diazepam and lorazepam, are sometimes used in addition to other medicines to help relieve restlessness, anxiety, panic or insomnia. They may allow lower doses of other medicines to be used. Unlike all the other medications used to help control bipolar disorder, the benzodiazepines are potentially addictive with long-term use. You may need increasingly high doses over time to get the same effect, and may experience symptoms of withdrawal when stopping them. This can be avoided if they are used only for short periods, and are used 'as needed' rather than regularly.

Electroconvulsive therapy

Although it is not a first-line treatment, electroconvulsive therapy (ECT) is an effective treatment for severe bipolar episodes. It tends to be used when other treatments have not been effective, or when there are substantial risks to the person, such as marked suicidal ideas. It is used predominantly for depression, but can treat other phases of the illness as well. For some people it can be a lifesaver. It involves giving an electrical stimulation to the brain under the use of an anaesthetic. People can experience some loss of memory or confusion around the period of the treatment.

Other adjunctive therapies

As an add-on to mood stabilisers, omega-3 fatty acids are of value for some people. Newer add-on therapies such as the antioxidant N-acetyl cysteine show promise, particularly for depression. Certain forms of psychotherapy used in addition to medication have been shown to reduce relapse in bipolar disorder (Colom et al., 2003b). Psychotherapy is discussed in the next chapter.

KEY POINTS

- Knowledge of your medical treatment can help you to make informed choices about treatment.
- In this chapter, we have discussed the different medications used to treat bipolar disorder and their use in the different phases of illness and in ongoing treatment.
- This chapter is an introduction to treatment options, and it may be useful to address questions and seek out more information from your doctor.
- Fortunately, medical treatment for bipolar disorder is a growing area and it is useful to keep up to date with the new research.

8 PSYCHOTHERAPY

Psychotherapy heals. It makes some sense of the confusion, reins in the terrifying thoughts and feelings, returns some control and hope and possibility of learning from it all . . . No pill can help me deal with the problem of not wanting to take pills; likewise, no amount of psychotherapy alone can prevent my manias and depressions. I need both.

Kay Jamison, *An Unquiet Mind*, 1997:89.

There is a growing body of evidence that supports the use of psychological interventions in conjunction with medication in the treatment of bipolar disorder. This chapter briefly introduces the different types of therapy that can be useful, and provides a broad guide to therapy.

WHAT IS PSYCHOTHERAPY?

'Psychotherapy' refers to a process that uses techniques and strategies designed to enhance a person's life and wellbeing. Psychotherapy is sometimes called 'talk therapy', a term which suggests a rather passive process and belies the effort involved in working through a particular issue or concern. Psychotherapy is not a replacement for medication, nor is it a cure for bipolar disorder, but it can help you make positive changes. What is involved varies according to the different types of psychotherapy and the needs of each person. A few specific types of therapy have been found helpful in managing bipolar disorder.

HOW CAN PSYCHOTHERAPY HELP?

Seeing a therapist can help you to:

- understand your bipolar disorder and find ways of treating it
- identify and manage triggers and early warning signs of illness, which will give you more control over the illness
- develop relapse prevention plans
- reduce symptoms of depression and anxiety
- talk through your problems and reduce stress
- get back on your feet after an episode of illness and deal with some of the consequences that can ensue from your mood swings
- develop a healthy lifestyle
- come to terms with your bipolar disorder and work out ways of leading a fulfilling life.

As Mark commented: 'It is like I now have a toolbox of things I can use that help, and I have them with me all the time. Which one I use and when will depend on how things are going for me.'

Often a specific issue or concern prompts a visit to a therapist. It might be that a recent episode of illness has been particularly disruptive and resulted in relationship or work problems, or has prompted a desire to find out more about the disorder, how it affects you and what can help to prevent relapse. Specific worries or concerns, around issues such as whether you should tell your colleagues that you have the disorder, or conflict with your partner, may be the reason for starting the process.

DIFFERENT TYPES OF THERAPY

There are a number of different types of therapy used in addition to medication for bipolar disorder. The goals of psychotherapy are to help you keep well and to prevent or reduce relapse and its consequences, as well as to enrich the quality of your life. While each perspective approaches this goal in a slightly different way, they all emphasise a collaboration between you and the therapist, highlighting information about bipolar disorder and the importance of knowing your moods, triggers and warning symptoms.

Psychoeducation

The major emphasis in psychoeducational approaches is on providing information about bipolar disorder and its treatment. Most psychotherapy approaches to bipolar disorder include some aspects of psychoeducation highlighting key aspects, such as:

- types of bipolar disorder and course of illness
- role of stress and triggers and early identification of warning signs
- medication
- positive ways of coping such as a healthy lifestyle, stress management and problem-solving strategies.

John was recently diagnosed with bipolar disorder and his doctor thought that some individual therapy sessions using a psychoeducational approach would be helpful. At his first session, his therapist, Paul, showed him a number of different graphs highlighting the mood fluctuations in different types of bipolar disorder. John was able to discuss with Paul how his experience of the illness fitted with this information. It made a lot more sense as John had not been aware of the different types of bipolar and had become very confused by some of the things he had read. Paul also reviewed the causes of bipolar, highlighting the biological and stress components. From this, he was able to demonstrate to John that there was scope for him to manage his illness, and they discussed strategies for preventing relapse.

Group psychoeducation has shown good results in reducing bipolar relapses, and psychoeducation may also be offered on an individual, couple or family basis (Colom et al., 2003a; Simon et al., 2006, Castle et al., 2007). Psychoeducation that focuses on helping people identify and respond to warning symptoms has been found to reduce manic relapse (Perry et al., 1999).

Cognitive and cognitive behavioural therapy

Cognitive therapy (CT) and cognitive behavioural therapy (CBT) are based on the relationship of thoughts (cognitions) and behaviour (the things you do) to the way you feel. The cornerstone of this approach is to alter particular thought patterns and beliefs that can negatively change behaviour and increase the risk of developing or worsening your mood.

Figure 8.1 demonstrates that the way we think and act can affect the way we feel. The diagram shows Claire's thinking pattern when George does not return an email.

From figure 8.1 we can see how unhelpful Claire's thoughts are. Her automatic response is that George doesn't like her, although there is little evidence to support this conclusion. Claire changes her behaviour because she feels down. She doesn't play her usual social game of tennis, which she enjoys. In doing this she removes an opportunity not only to enjoy the game of tennis but also to receive other positive input from her friends.

The unpleasant feelings (sadness and rejection) can be mediated by changing what occurs at either of the other two points, the levels of thought or behaviour. Look what happens in figure 8.2 if Claire changes her thoughts and realises that George may be very busy and that is why he is not replying, or if she responds to the unpleasant feelings by going to play tennis, which she enjoys (her behaviour).

The topics of a CT or CBT program vary depending on the needs of the individual, but generally include similar elements to

Figure 8.1 Negative thinking

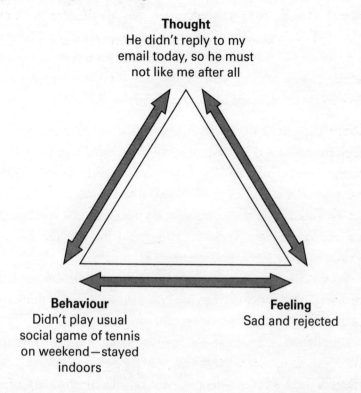

Thought
He didn't reply to my
email today, so he must
not like me after all

Behaviour
Didn't play usual
social game of tennis
on weekend—stayed
indoors

Feeling
Sad and rejected

a psychoeducational approach, with a focus on learning and applying skills and strategies. There are additional elements such as learning about unhelpful thinking and how to monitor and change it, and developing relapse prevention plans. Some people with bipolar disorder find that changing behaviour may be even more helpful than changing their thinking when they are becoming depressed or manic (see chapters 11 and 14).

In between each session, clients are usually asked to complete 'homework' tasks which are discussed in the next session. The 'homework' provides an opportunity to practise skills taught in the sessions. Attention is also paid to sorting out realistic problems that are a source of concern to the client.

Figure 8.2 Changing thinking and behaviour

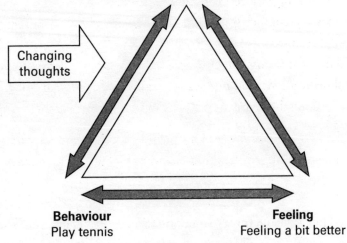

Alternative thought
*There could be a number of reasons why
he may not have replied to my email
today—perhaps he had a very busy day*

Changing
thoughts

Behaviour
Play tennis

Feeling
Feeling a bit better

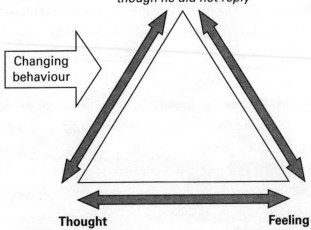

Alternative behaviour
*Decide to play tennis even
though he did not reply*

Changing
behaviour

Thought
He didn't reply to my email
but there are a number of
possible reasons for this
that I can check out

Feeling
Felt bad initially but
had a good game
with friends and lifted
my mood a bit

Family-focused therapy

Family-focused therapy is an inclusive approach that involves the person with bipolar disorder as well as members of their family (Miklowitz et al., 2003). The aim is to strengthen healthy interaction and support between family members and to help resolve any existing conflict in the family. The family works together to prevent relapse.

This form of therapy has three major components: psychoeducation, communication skills and problem solving. This is done through family discussions.

- The *psychoeducation* sessions provide family members with an understanding of the disorder and its biological nature, as well as the influence of stressors, and of coping strategies.
- The *communication* sessions encourage positive feedback and counter dysfunctional communication styles, which are seen as a sign of the family's struggle to cope with the disorder. Family members role-play active listening and making positive requests (see chapter 19).
- *Problem-solving* is the tool this approach uses to teach families how to deal with difficulties and disagreements. Together family members identify and assess possible solutions and develop a plan of action.

Family-focused therapy has also been used to deal with the issue of suicide, taking the approach that suicidal feelings are a part of the illness. Openly talking about these feelings with family members and developing a joint suicide prevention plan can help you gain control over these distressing thoughts and feelings and prevent suicide.

Interpersonal and social rhythm therapy

Interpersonal and social rhythm therapy (IPSRT) builds on an existing therapy known as interpersonal therapy (IPT) (Frank,

2007). IPSRT emphasises the role of interpersonal relationships on mental wellbeing. It recognises the role of loss and grief in dealing with bipolar disorder, and offers clients the opportunity to express this and develop personal ways of adjusting.

The other key element of IPSRT in dealing with bipolar disorder relates to the patterns of daily life, our *social rhythms*. This approach emphasises how a disruption to regular social rhythms can trigger an episode of illness. There is evidence that regular day–night (circadian) rhythms are important in maintaining stable mood in bipolar disorder. The patterns of daily life include such things as the time we get up and go to bed, and our usual activities, such as going to work or a regular morning meeting with friends. People involved in this therapy are encouraged to monitor their sleep/wake cycle (circadian rhythm), patterns of daily activity and levels of daily stimulation, like the number of people they come into contact with. This allows them to regulate their daily patterns so their mood is not disrupted.

Michelle, a 30-year-old single woman, now works from home as a freelance journalist. Michelle realised that since her first episode of bipolar disorder there had been many changes in her life. She had changed her job and had lost some of her friends who did not understand what she was going through. In therapy she realised that she was grieving for the things she had lost. She actually enjoyed her current job and realised that there were a few people she had met at work and through her local support group who were keen to be friends, as well as one or two people from the past. She had previously avoided social arrangements because she still felt so hurt about her lost friendships. Her therapist helped her take steps to connect with some of these people. Looking at a timeline of her illness, they discovered that Michelle's episodes of illness seemed to be associated with meeting a story deadline, which usually meant she had stayed up late a number of nights in a row to try to get it in. Her therapist helped her understand more about bipolar disorder and what can trigger an episode. She also introduced Michelle to monitoring her social rhythms so that any changes could quickly be acted upon. Michelle found that monitoring had the added bonus of helping her to maintain a flexible routine.

BEGINNING THERAPY

The therapy approach can vary depending on personal preference. Some approaches may be more suited to particular individuals— for example, family-focused approaches would be appropriate in the context of obvious problems within a family. However, beginning therapy is not just about the approach, it is also about choosing the right therapist. As with your relationship with your doctor, having a good working relationship with your therapist is essential, and it might be necessary to see more than one person initially to make the choice.

Tips for starting psychotherapy

- Ask your doctor, friends or consumer groups to recommend a therapist.
- Psychological societies have 'find a psychologist' sections on their websites, which can help you find a therapist in your area.
- It is always worth checking that the person you are planning to see is appropriately qualified and registered and has some experience in working with people with bipolar disorder.
- You can enquire what sort of perspective they tend to use when working with clients, for example, cognitive therapy or a family approach.
- You may want to know how many sessions you will need. This can be difficult to quantify; however, there should be a set review point at which you and the therapist evaluate how things have been going. Sometimes the number of sessions is limited by the financial cost.

- Establishing regular times for appointments can make them fit in with your routine and make them easier to remember.
- Do not be afraid to discuss cost. The cost of therapy varies widely so it is worth checking what yours will cost and whether it is covered by your health insurance scheme.
- It is important that the therapy is relevant to you at that time. It may be that you are dealing with a number of issues as well as bipolar disorder. If you are about to be evicted from your home, or are in the middle of a divorce, you are unlikely to pay much attention to a therapy session intended to explore the warning signs of illness. At these times, issues beyond bipolar illness may need to be made a more prominent focus of the sessions.
- It might be helpful to clarify what problems you want to address or what goals you want to achieve—for example, learning strategies to prevent relapse or dealing with a problematic relationship. This can help you to work out what you want to get out of psychotherapy. You can always return at a later stage if you wish to address other issues.

ANOTHER DIRECTION

Mindfulness-based cognitive therapy (MBCT) includes meditative techniques through which people are taught to become aware of sensations, thoughts and feelings, and to change their typical automatic responses to them. For people who have experienced a number of unipolar depressive episodes, these techniques may be useful in managing depressive thoughts and feelings (Segal et al., 2002). The applicability of this approach to bipolar disorder is being examined by researchers.

KEY POINTS

- A number of different psychological approaches can be useful in managing bipolar illness when combined with medication. These include:

- psychoeducation
- cognitive and cognitive behavioural therapy
- family-focused therapy.
- interpersonal and social rhythm therapy
- The strategies offered by these perspectives have some key common themes such as information about the disorder and medication, triggers of illness and developing strategies to minimise relapse.
- There are, however, some key differences of particular therapeutic approaches, but no specific therapy approach has been found to be superior.
- You can use the recommendations of your doctor and others whose opinions you value to help you find a therapist who suits you.
- There are a number of useful tips to help you get started in psychotherapy.

9 MANAGING YOUR TRIGGERS

I believe that only a part of managing my bipolar disorder is about putting out the fire and dealing with the symptoms. An important part is also managing those stressful things that trigger my symptoms. Sure, it puts some limitations on my life, but it also gives me greater freedom to enjoy my relationships, work and the things I value in life. **Sue**

Identifying stressful triggers and finding ways of responding to them to help prevent relapse is a strategy used by many people with bipolar disorder. Stress is actually a physical response involving changes in the body in order to adapt to the demands of a situation. Not all stress is bad, however, and life is full of challenges and opportunities through which we grow and achieve. Stress becomes a problem when there is too much of it, when a certain type of stress is particularly upsetting for you or when you are not well enough to deal with it. Experiencing such stress not only feels bad, it can also compromise biological functions, such as immunity and the production of certain hormones, and it affects the brain's neurotransmitters. These may be the paths through which stress affects your health. Becoming familiar with the triggers of your bipolar disorder and finding ways of reducing them can give you more control over your illness.

STRESSFUL EVENTS

Stressful events are a part of life. People often think of stressful events as those difficult negative life events or major changes that everyone is confronted with from time to time, such as a death in the family, losing a job, moving house or the end of a relationship. Stressful life events can also be big positive changes, such as getting married, having a baby, beginning a romantic relationship, passing an exam or being promoted.

Sometimes the few weeks after an episode of illness can be stressful if a person is confronted with some of the consequences resulting from their illness, and accumulated demands. Sometimes moods are triggered by minor events, such as having someone come to stay, or a dose of the flu. You may also find that it is not one event but the accumulation of a number of minor or major events that triggers an episode of illness.

Emotions can run high when we encounter both positive and negative stressful events. Strategies which can help guard against relapse at these times include such things as re-establishing regular sleep habits, routines and activity levels that may have been disrupted by the event, doing relaxing and soothing activities and expressing your feelings in a journal or through art or music. Talking things through with a trusted person and keeping an extra eye out for your typical warning symptoms can also help. Keeping expectations of yourself realistic and prioritising tasks may reduce pressure when you are confronted with a stressful event. Taking things one day at a time and getting support from a counsellor can reduce stress (see chapter 18).

The way you think

The way you think about an event may influence how stressful you find it. For example, if you think that a particular event is a catastrophe over which you have no control, you may experience extreme stress, which could influence your mood. On the other hand, you could see the same event as unfortunate and feel upset, but believe that you will get through it and find ways to solve the problems it causes. Challenging negative thinking and putting things into perspective can be useful in allowing you to move forward and deal with the stress (see chapter 12). Problem solving is a useful skill to reduce the stress of negative events (see chapter 18 and the website associated with this book).

Your moods

People who already have mild mood symptoms may be more susceptible to stressful events (Johnson, 2005). Assuming the worst, and having little energy or confidence, which are typical symptoms of depression, can make even good things seem overwhelming and make it harder to deal with stressful demands or events. Likewise, if you are a bit hypomanic, you may see such events as challenges, and become increasingly busy and sleep deprived and hypomanic as you strive to meet the challenge. Treating your mild or early symptoms may make you less vulnerable to stress.

> The build-up to opening night of my plays and the celebrations afterwards make me dizzy with success. My thoughts start to race, and it is hard to sleep. I have learnt that if I take the extra medication prescribed by my doctor for these times, limit the hours of celebration and try to maintain my basic routine, particularly sleep, I can enjoy these times without becoming manic.
> **Pam**

SLEEP, STIMULATION AND ACTIVITY LEVELS

People with bipolar disorder are thought to be particularly sensitive to changes in their sleep/wake cycle and to changes in the amount of stimulation they get from social activity, work and daily routines.

Routine and structure

Social rhythms are those patterns of everyday activity—falling asleep, waking up, having meals and social interaction—that structure daily life and set your body clock. Doing some things routinely may help regulate sleep/wake cycles. People with bipolar disorder are sensitive to changes in social rhythms, which can act as stressors to trigger symptoms. If disruptions affect your sleep/wake cycle, you may need to problem solve around them to prevent them from triggering relapse.

You can draw up a weekly timetable to try to keep your social rhythms relatively stable so they do not affect your mood. Including the things you plan to do, time off to act spontaneously and your usual activity and sleep patterns in this timetable may help keep your mood stable. It can also be useful to use your timetable to regulate your sleep and activity level if you notice symptoms of illness. We call this timetable the Mood and Activity Schedule; it is explained in chapter 16.

The way you respond to disruption to your activity levels or sleep is important. For example, say, you have just got a promotion and are feeling really excited so you celebrate and don't get much sleep. If you feel wound up and see the promotion as proof of your importance, and so take on more at work, carry on celebrating and sleep less, you might wind up hypomanic or manic. On the other hand, once you have celebrated you could try returning to your routine and restoring your sleep as soon as possible to prevent your mood from escalating further.

Sensitivity to stimulation

People with bipolar disorder can be sensitive to even minor changes in stimulation especially when they are a bit sympto-matic. For example, a cluttered or messy house, noise, traffic, lots of activity going on around you, time pressures or extra social stimulation may increase symptoms of hypomania, mania or mixed states or even depression. In Jody's case: 'The summer sales make me feel hyped up and overstimulated, and I spend much too much money. I need to unwind and do very relaxing, quiet activities when I get home or I continue to race.' Depression may also be connected to under-stimulation, such as having little social contact, lack of light over winter months, lack of structure and doing nothing.

Knowing what affects your mood can help you to regulate your level of stimulation. For example, you can try and reduce clutter and noise if these are very stimulating, and maintain regular activity levels when on holiday to avoid becoming overstimulated.

Chasing goals

Sometimes chasing your goals can lead to overstimulation. Many people with bipolar disorder find that keeping well requires them to adjust their goals and the way they pursue them. If your goals are causing too much stress and disrupting your usual patterns, it may be helpful to check if they are realistic (see the SMART goal setting tool on this book's website) and to increase the period you've allowed for achieving them. Turn the goals you want to achieve soon into more long-term goals; in other words, give yourself more time to achieve them without things becoming too stressful. Prioritise goals into high, medium and low priority, so you don't feel as though you have to achieve everything at once. Delegate the things you don't have to do yourself. Choosing not to take on too much can reduce your stress levels. In addition, you could look for alternative goals that will still allow you to express your strengths and talents but are less likely to trigger your illness (see chapter 18). This might involve finding creative compromises that are realistic and fit with your values and priorities.

Sometimes it is not the goals themselves that are the problem, but rather the way you are trying to achieve them. Pursuing goals in a structured way that does not disrupt your basic routine or sleep patterns may take more time, but it can mean that you stay well and complete things. Organising your goals into 'goal steps' which you include in your Mood and Activity Schedule can help to achieve this (see chapter 16).

Good sleep habits

At times it can be difficult to avoid sleep disruptions—holidays, family commitments and high work demands can often put pressure on your sleep/wake routine. Despite such difficulties, it is important to keep to a flexible routine so that any disruption is kept to a minimum. There are a number of things you can do to help get a good night's sleep (Erman, 2005). Here are some tips:

- Keep your bedroom clear of stimulation such as noise or lights. People tend to sleep better in a cooler environment, so turn down the thermostat. Keeping the bedroom as a special place for sleeping or intimacy helps your body and mind relax because you come to associate going to bed with these things.
- Try not to do things that are very stimulating—like work, lively discussions or an argument—just before going to sleep.
- Avoid caffeine, which is found in coffee, cola drinks and chocolate, for at least eight hours before bedtime. Although many people attest that caffeine doesn't affect their sleep, research has clearly shown that even for those who 'don't feel as if it affects them', it does. Caffeine is thought to block adenosine, the body's natural sleep-producing chemical. Following the ingestion of caffeine, people take longer to fall asleep, and their quality of sleep is also changed.
- Having alcohol within six hours before bedtime can also reduce the quality of your sleep. With long-term use of alcohol, the body adapts by being more anxious and wakeful.

To improve your sleep you may need to reduce your alcohol consumption.

- Although smoking is best avoided completely for your health, it is particularly important to avoid smoking for at least two hours before bed due to the stimulating properties of nicotine.
- Daytime naps can make it harder to fall asleep, and can decrease the quality of your sleep. If you have difficulty sleeping at night, don't try to catch up by sleeping more at other times (sleep bingeing), as this will make it even harder to restore your sleep routine. Rather, stop the daytime sleep and try to restore your regular sleep and wake times.
- Take care in when you schedule exercise. A regular exercise program during the day can increase the depth of sleep, but exercise just before sleep can make sleeping more difficult. It is thought this is due to an increase in temperature in body and brain.
- Put your bedside clock out of view so you can't 'clock watch' during the night.
- Going to bed very hungry can disturb sleep. A light snack at bedtime, such as a glass of warm milk, can be helpful. On the other hand, a heavy meal too late in the evening can also disturb sleep.
- Try to keep to a routine of going to bed and getting up around the same time each day. This helps your body to develop a regular time of going to sleep. Your day–night internal clock is mainly set by daylight, and waking at a consistent time every morning is the most important part of this routine. There will be periods when the times you wake up and go to sleep are unavoidably disrupted; the important thing here is to return to your regular sleep/wake times as soon as you can. Even when you don't get to sleep at your usual time, try to get up at your usual time. Keep to your sleep/wake times even if events change, for example, on holiday.

- Developing a 'wind-down' routine before you go to bed can signal to your body that it is time to go to sleep. This can involve a relaxing activity such as reading, having a warm bath or listening to music. Proper relaxation exercises, such as progressive muscle relaxation and breathing techniques, done when you get into bed, can also calm you down (see chapter 18). For some people, thinking of a peaceful scene and imagining they are there and at peace can help them relax and fall asleep.

Two forms of worry can intrude on getting to sleep.

- The first is thoughts about things in your day that seem to demand attention as soon as your head hits the pillow. It can help to write a 'worry list' of these daytime worries to deal with the next day, and to give yourself permission to put these worries on hold.
- The other type of worry thoughts are those about sleep itself. It might be worry about how long it will take to go to sleep or, if you wake during the night, worry about not being able to get back to sleep. For example, 'Oh heck, it's 2 a.m. and I'm still awake. I must get to sleep immediately . . . If I don't get to sleep now, tomorrow will be such a disaster and I just know I won't cope.' It can help to let yourself off the hook, to reassure yourself that you will deal with things tomorrow, meanwhile focusing on relaxing, rather than trying to sleep. Reassuring self-talk can help: 'Oh, I'm still awake. OK, I don't feel good about still being awake. For now I will concentrate on just relaxing, and in the morning I'll make an appointment to see my doctor so this problem can be nipped in the bud.'
- If after some time you still cannot sleep, get up, go into another room and do some relaxing activity, like listening to soothing music, then return to bed. Do *not* engage in any stimulating activity such as surfing the net, housework or

watching an exciting movie. The idea is to do something quiet, boring and calming.

As sleep disturbance can be a warning sign or an early symptom of bipolar illness, it is useful to talk to your doctor about using medication as a temporary measure to restore your sleep patterns.

Jet lag can disrupt sleep habits. If you have to travel to a later time zone and you will be there for more than a few days, try, over the course of the week before you travel, to go to bed an hour earlier than usual, then a hour and a half, two hours earlier, and so on. This will help you adjust more gradually to the time change. Once you arrive, stick to regular sleep habits appropriate to that time zone. Don't rush around getting too overstimulated in the day.

INTERPERSONAL CONFLICT

All relationships have their ups and downs, and the symptoms and consequences of bipolar disorder can place stress on relationships. Some people are particularly sensitive to interpersonal conflict and rejection, especially if they already have mild symptoms. If those close to you are critical, hostile or over-protective and this is distressing for you, this stress may increase the risk of relapse.

Common sense tells us that other types of interpersonal conflict, such as conflicts at work, might also act as triggers of illness. If you consider that you may be seeing things in a one-sided, negative light, using the Helpful Thought Summary in chapter 12 may help you to put the situation into perspective. The skills explained in chapter 19 might also assist you in sorting out disagreements and conflicts.

DRUGS AND ALCOHOL

Around half the people with bipolar disorder abuse alcohol or drugs, which makes their illness worse and leads to more hospital admissions. No one really knows why there is such a strong link between drug and alcohol problems and bipolar disorder. For many individuals the mood disorder predates the substance use disorder. Because of this it is thought that people who have both bipolar disorder and drug or alcohol problems tend to use these substances in an attempt to 'treat' the symptoms of their disorder. In the long run, however, drugs and alcohol significantly worsen mood in people who have bipolar disorder.

The key to understanding the problematic effects of such substances is that the body will always adapt to the presence of any substance by 'going the other way', to restore its usual balance or homeostasis, in the same way that if one drinks too much water the body reacts by increasing urine output. What this means is that with a substance like alcohol you may initially experience a positive shift in mood from having a few drinks, such as feeling sleepy and relaxed, but then your body adapts by reducing your positive mood, so you feel worse with time, and need more and more alcohol to get the desired effect. As you become more dependent on alcohol you may find it harder to stop drinking, because being off alcohol makes you feel anxious and unable to sleep, so you become stuck in a vicious cycle that makes your mood worse. Similarly, amphetamines cause an initial high with an increase in energy, but their long-term use can lead to depression and lethargy. Marijuana use can lead to apathy, depression, sleep disruption, anxiety and psychotic symptoms. Cocaine and hallucinogens can trigger illness episodes and more hospital admissions.

In addition, substance abuse decreases the chances of responding well to medications prescribed for bipolar disorder (Singh & Zarate, 2006). You may believe that it is only the more serious street drugs that worsen the illness, but research currently in progress shows that smokers also have more relapses and might not respond well to treatment (Berk, 2007).

Sometimes people take drugs to seek out hypomania. Steve, a 30-year-old financial consultant with bipolar I disorder, explains his encounter with drugs. His heavy drug use started with the success of his business:

> I found that as my business was growing, it was becoming more difficult to find time to attend to all my clients. I reasoned that if I took speed daily I might feel just hypomanic enough to get through the workload. I found I needed less sleep and initially had more energy, but I also began to feel increasingly irritable and paranoid, had racing thoughts and was becoming so agitated that I was finding it hard to complete tasks. As the speed wore off, most of these symptoms persisted, but I also felt exhausted. My wife and kids were upset by my explosive outbursts, and my clients were angry, as I was not delivering on my promises. I started feeling desperate as my relationships and career were falling apart. I called my doctor and was admitted to hospital as a voluntary patient. I plan to stay off speed and to try to develop a healthier lifestyle. It just wasn't worth it.

For many people, even when they know that alcohol or drugs are making them more ill, it can be hard to decide to do something about it. A good idea is to look at the pros and cons of your current substance use in terms of what is really important to you, and your personal goals and values, to help you decide.

If you decide to try to break this habit, it is useful to do so in collaboration with your clinician and key support people. Some helpful resources are listed on www.eburypublishing. co.uk/bipolar.

PHYSICAL ILLNESS

Some people with bipolar illness have found that physical illness, for example an infection, acts as a stressor and affects their mood. The reasons behind physical illness affecting mood include biological explanations as well as the disruption to normal routines and activities. Seeing your doctor and having the physical illness treated as quickly as possible can help limit the time you are unwell and reduce its impact on your mood.

At times, it can be hard to distinguish the symptoms of a physical illness and mood. Having a bad cold, for example, can make you feel lethargic and just want to stay in bed all day. Monitoring both your mood and your cold symptoms, and discussing the issue with your doctor, can help you to consider when it would be best to return to your usual routine.

STOPPING HELPFUL MEDICATIONS

Sometimes side effects make it necessary to change medications even though it has helped your mood. Stopping a medication that is having a beneficial effect on your mood can be a powerful trigger of illness. You can weigh up the pros and cons of taking the medication and discuss this with your clinician before making such a decision.

SEASONAL HIGH RISK

The better you can predict your high-risk times, the better you can prepare yourself to manage your illness at these times and reduce the likelihood of relapse. Knowing your triggers not only provides the opportunity to reduce them if they arise, it is also a signal to observe whether warning symptoms are developing so that you can act to prevent or reduce relapse.

Identifying a pattern of illness connected to the seasons, or a tendency to cycle from one particular phase of illness into another, can also be helpful. Knowing that these are high-risk times can mean taking extra precautions, such as regulating your sleep and activity levels and making regular check-up appointments with your doctor.

Some people report finding it helpful to spend time under bright lights if the darker months trigger depression. This so-called 'bright light therapy' has been used to treat seasonal affective disorder in people suffering from unipolar depression. Because people with bipolar disorder are sensitive to stimulation, it would be best to discuss such strategies with your clinician before attempting them.

DISCOVERING YOUR TRIGGERS

Not all episodes of bipolar disorder have identifiable triggers, but some do. Being able to identify triggers of the different phases of illness allows people to work out strategies to include in their plans to prevent or at least to minimise relapse (chapter 17). Here are some tips for discovering your triggers.

Know yourself

An event may be particularly stressful if it affects an important area of your life. For example, if you are socially oriented you may be harder hit by events or conflicts that threaten relationships. If achievement and high standards of performance are of central importance to you, it might be events affecting these areas that trigger symptoms.

Considering your personality may give you more clues about the sorts of situations or events that you find stressful. For example, a perfectionist may be more vulnerable when regular daily events don't run according to plan (Scott, 2001).

Track previous episodes

'Life charting' is a tool that involves reflecting on times of wellness and illness and working out whether particular episodes were sparked off by particular triggers. Episodes are recorded on a timeline that roughly indicates the date and duration of the episode, as well as the type of relapse.

Figure 9.1a Drawing your life chart

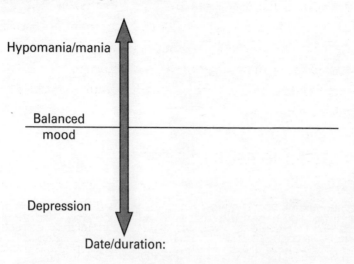

The life chart (see figures 9.1 a and b) includes:

* approximate date or year and duration of episode
* type of episode (mania, hypomania, depression or mixed)
* periods of wellbeing
* possible triggers.

The midway horizontal line represents times of 'normal' balanced mood. What is above the line represents hypomania and mania, and below the line, depression. The idea is to draw curves as shown in Wendy's example (figure 9.2) to represent your episodes of illness. The higher the curve, the more severe the symptoms, and the wider the curve, the longer the episode's duration. To indicate mixed episodes you can place corresponding curves above and below the line (see figure 9.1b).

On the line at the base of the chart is space for the rough date or period of the episode. Recalling what age you were at the time, or what else was happening in your life, may help to work out time frames.

If you have only recently been diagnosed, you may feel you don't have much to chart, but if you think back to before your

Figure 9.1b Mixed episode

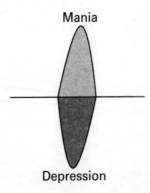

Mania

Depression

diagnosis, you may realise that you had earlier mood swings that were not recognised at the time. If you have been diagnosed for a number of years, you may find it easier to start with noting your most recent episode and working backwards.

Once you have noted your mood episodes on the chart, and their date and duration, the next step is to add triggers. These include major events such as the beginning or end of a relationship, moving house, birth of a child, as well as the other possible triggers discussed earlier in this chapter that might have occurred around the time of an episode. A trusted friend may be helpful in recalling triggers and episodes of illness. A blank life chart is available for your personal use on the website associated with this book.

Example of a life chart

Figure 9.2 shows Wendy's life chart. Her first episode occurred when she finished high school. She experienced a brief period of hypomania (ten days) followed by a depressive episode lasting about four months. She started university in 1996, and things were going well until another episode in 1999 that occurred after her exams. Wendy recalled she had stopped taking her medication at that time. This episode was more severe than the first one. Her elevated mood was higher, and it was followed by a slightly longer period of depression. In reflecting on her life chart, Wendy was

Figure 9.2 Wendy's life chart

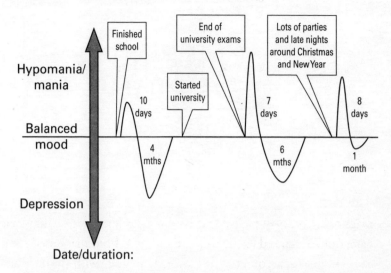

aware that at the end of her exams she tended to party a lot and forget her medication. The same thing happened a year later when she increased her social activity at Christmas time. She realised that a high level of social activity was a major trigger of illness and that she might need to moderate her social activity a bit and be sure to take her medications at such times.

KEY POINTS

- Certain stressors may trigger your vulnerability to developing a specific type of mood episode.
- These triggers include stressful events, sleep and activity disruption, sensitivity to stimulation, chasing goals, interpersonal conflict, drug and alcohol problems, physical illness, stopping helpful medication, the seasons, and high risk due to cycling from one mood to another.
- Knowing what may trigger your moods can help you to find responses that reduce the risk of relapse at these times.
- You can include your ideas for managing triggers in your plans to prevent relapse.

10 CATCHING SYMPTOMS EARLY

One of the things that has made a huge difference to living with my bipolar is that I have learnt to recognise the signs that I am becoming ill and to get treatment early. When they do occur, my moods are less extreme and cause less disruption to my life. **Frank**

Many people with bipolar disorder find that controlling their medications and managing triggers is part of a healthy lifestyle that helps keep them well. It is still a good idea to be prepared to prevent or reduce relapse if symptoms do arise. Of course, severe symptoms can be treated, but catching them early gives you a chance to prevent or reduce the severity or duration of an episode of illness. It also means that you can prepare to reduce the potentially damaging consequences of episodes in case things get worse. This way you have an extra buffer against the effects of relapse.

It is important to be mindful of changes in how you behave, feel or think that signal you are becoming ill, not just as a matter of curiosity, but to gain more control over your bipolar disorder. 'Prodromes' are signs and symptoms that precede and lead up to the point at which an episode of illness is at its most severe (Molnar et al., 1988). If you can identify warning or early symptoms of illness, you can take action to reduce relapse. There are ideas for ways of responding to these warnings and early symptoms in the following chapters.

A RELAPSE SIGNATURE

In the same way as you have particular triggers of illness to which you are more sensitive, you may also have your own pattern of how warning signs and symptoms develop into a specific type of episode (mania, hypomania, depression or mixed states). This is called a 'relapse signature' (Lam et al., 2001). Recognising your relapse signature can take time, especially if you have had only a single episode of illness. Some people do not have a stable relapse signature, and they find it more helpful to know the typical symptoms of the various types of episode and to keep their eyes open for these more general early signs.

Most people with bipolar disorder are able to identify warning symptoms of mania (Lam & Wong, 1997), although people who experience mild symptoms between episodes sometimes find it hard to work out when these end and warning symptoms appear. Often it is when these symptoms become more intense, or new symptoms develop, that they realise they are developing warning signs. It is easier to identify warning symptoms of mania than of depression. Warning symptoms of depression may be more subtle and harder to distinguish from the mild symptoms that sometimes persist between episodes. Some people may notice symptoms of depression only when an episode has already begun, but catching them early and intervening effectively may still make a difference.

COMMON AND UNIQUE PRODROMES

People experience many different prodromes when they are becoming ill, and the idea is to find those that are typical for you and that you can identify as early as possible when you are becoming ill. These may be prodromes that are commonly experienced or those that are unique signs of your own. Although many other symptoms may be experienced as prodromes, the most common are listed below.

Common prodromes of mania and hypomania

The most common warning symptoms of mania are:

- reduced sleep
- doing lots more activities and having more energy
- being more sociable
- irritability
- racing thoughts
- increased self-confidence, self-importance and optimism
- heightened senses (Lam & Wong, 2006).

People with bipolar II sometimes find it hard to distinguish prodromes from their usual mood. Common prodromes these people may notice when becoming hypomanic are slight sleep reduction, raised energy levels, increased speed of thinking or speech, irritability and impatience (Miklowitz, 2002).

Other prodromes that are often reported when people are becoming hypomanic or manic are:

- new ideas, plans or interests
- risky driving or other risky activities
- increased sex drive.

Common prodromes of depression

The most common prodromes of depression are:

- losing interest or enjoyment in activities or people
- persistent worry or anxiety
- sleep disruption
- feeling sad and tearful (Lam & Wong, 2006).

Other prodromes that are often reported include:

- neglect of tasks and reduction in activities
- fatigue
- physical aches
- being forgetful
- social withdrawal.

If you experience mixed episodes, you may have prodromes that are typical of either mania or depression or a mixture of prodromes from both types of episode.

Unique prodomes

Here are some examples of more unusual early warnings:

> I know when I am becoming manic as I wear more makeup than usual and change my hair colour more often and I wear shorter skirts and more revealing outfits. **Talia**

> A symptom of going down for me is that I lose my sense of taste. All food starts to taste the same, and then I just can't be bothered to eat. **Kalib**

Often you may find that your personal warning signs are excellent very early clues; you may develop other more typical symptoms as later warning symptoms before your episode starts.

> I always thought my depressions just hit me like a steam train with no warning but I have found a very early sign and a few slightly later symptoms to use in my relapse prevention plan. I pride myself on doing the crossword every night. A very early sign is when I just can't find the right words to fill in so it takes much longer. The next thing is finding it harder to fall asleep. Instead I lie awake worrying about the next day even when nothing special is happening. During the day my 'zoom' has gone. A few weeks later everything goes dark and my depression has arrived. **Nick**

Looking for personal early signs, which are small changes that predate actual warning or early symptoms, can mean that you have a greater chance of catching and preventing an oncoming episode.

DEVELOPING YOUR PRODROME LIST

Identifying a few symptoms you typically experience before or at the start of each of the types of episodes you have can help you to gain more control over the course of your illness. It can be useful to write down the prodromal symptoms separately for each type of episode and to keep the list on hand so that you can recognise and respond to them in future. You can develop your own prodrome list on the website associated with this book. This list can become part of your action plan to reduce relapse and should be considered a work in progress. You may identify more early symptoms with time; with experience you can work out the most effective ways of responding to them to prevent or reduce an episode.

Here are some ideas for making it easier to identify and use your prodromes.

Get in early

People with bipolar disorder who have been well for at least two years say that some prodromal symptoms can be late rather than early warning symptoms (Russell, 2005). Once you have identified a warning or early symptom, dig a bit deeper and ask yourself if there is any change in the way you behave, feel or view things that may be a warning sign of that warning sign.

Learn from the past

Some people find it easy to recall previous episodes and how they developed, or to identify situations that arose before becoming ill, which helps them to identify their warning signs. The list of symptoms that typically form part of each of your episodes may help you to work out how these symptoms developed.

> I play tennis every week, and when I cancel a few consecutive tennis dates because I don't feel like going, I need to keep an eye on my mood to see if I am becoming depressed. I also start to worry about every little thing and neglect important chores like doing the washing. **Pam**

Before developing a mixed episode, I become very irritated with the mess around the house. My family very seldom worries about tidying things, and I become more irritable with them when I am going up. **Rennie**

Different to usual

Prodromes are different to how you usually feel, think or behave. It is important to distinguish warning symptoms from everyday ups and downs. Mood symptoms are more extreme, persistent and harder to shift, and have more consequences than everyday ups and downs, which are often reactions to events and subside soon afterwards. With everyday ups and downs it is generally easy to understand why you feel so happy or so sad. Mood symptoms are often unrelated or disproportional to external factors.

Enlist an extra pair of eyes

It can be helpful to ask someone who knows you well to help you identify your prodromes and draw up your prodrome list. Sometimes when people are becoming ill, part of the illness is failing to recognise their emerging symptoms. Those close to you might notice both minor and more major changes that signal warning signs, as in these examples:

My mum noticed that when I was going high, I started helping much more around the house and became much more talkative. I never even noticed this change. **Sara**

Jack usually eats a healthy diet, but when he goes and hunts for starch and sweet things after dinner for a week, and then just wants to go to sleep without even watching TV, he and I know to look for other symptoms of depression. **Emma**

Most easily noticeable prodromes

If possible, try to identify between three and six personal prodromes, then reduce the list to the few most easily noticeable signs for each type of episode. You may find that the easiest prodromes to spot are changes in what you do. For example, 'feeling a bit low' may not be as noticeable a sign as 'not bothering with my appearance' or 'cancelling lots of arrangements'. For other people changes in the way they see things or major changes in their thinking are also useful signs. Examples before becoming depressed include, 'Rather than my usual faith in my football team, I start seeing all their flaws and become convinced that they will lose' or 'I keep criticising myself'. Noticing obvious changes in how you feel, such as feeling more excited for no reason or more worried about everything, can be useful too. Sometimes being as specific as possible can help; instead of just listing 'sleep difficulties', include what those difficulties are, such as 'can't fall asleep at night' or 'wake up during the night and can't go back to sleep' or 'sleep during the day'.

If you have some of the same warning signs for, say, both depression and mania, such as loss of appetite or irritability, it can be helpful to make a mental note that these are messages telling you to pay attention to your illness. However, it is much more useful to find some specific warning signs for each type of episode.

Timelines

The duration of warning symptoms varies from person to person. It can be an extra advantage to know how far in advance of an episode symptoms begin to occur, or which symptoms develop early and which come later. This will enable you to decide how to respond to early symptoms, depending on how much time you have before things get worse. Monitoring these symptoms will give you an idea of when to put your various strategies to reduce relapse into place (see chapter 16). Some people cannot pinpoint things so precisely along the course of their illness, but it can still be useful to identify and respond to signs and symptoms as early as possible.

I asked my partner to help me recall the times when I become manic. We worked out that between episodes I am usually a bit hyped up and irritable. What changes is that I start phoning people and make lots of arrangements and this pleasant sociable time lasts for about two weeks. This is followed by an extra busy time where I feel extra confident and take on lots of projects. After another week, it becomes impossible to take breaks and my thoughts race. I stop sleeping and the mania really sets in. **Charlie**

KEY POINTS

- Catching changes in your thinking, feelings and behaviour as early as possible gives you a chance to prevent or at least reduce the severity of a full episode, and to minimise disruptive or dangerous consequences.

- Many people find it easier to identify warning signs or prodromes that occur when they are becoming hypomanic or manic than when they become depressed.

- There are common prodromes as well as more unique personal signs; some might be early warnings while others may occur closer to or at the start of your episode.

- Tips for identifying prodromes include learning from past experience; identifying noticeable changes from usual behaviours, and asking trusted others for their observations.

- It can be useful to have an idea of the timing and duration of early and late warning symptoms so that you can monitor how you are doing.

- A summary list of the typical warning or early symptoms for each type of episode you experience can be included in your plans to prevent or reduce relapse and prompt you to take action and implement constructive strategies if they occur.

11 SUPPORT AND ACTIVITY STRATEGIES WHEN BECOMING DEPRESSED

It was like falling into a deep pit, but now I realise that there is a rope around my waist and I can climb out. **Sam**

Catching and responding to warning or early symptoms of an episode of depression may help to prevent or reduce full episodes of illness. In addition to treating your depressive episodes with medication or a combination of medication and psychotherapy, you can use constructive self-management strategies to manage your warning or early symptoms, including:

- contacting your clinician and support network
- maintaining or restoring your activity level
- doing exercise and other enriching activities
- restoring your sleep habits
- putting pessimistic and undermining thinking in perspective and not making important decisions.

Strategies that have been reported to be unhelpful include 'doing nothing', staying in bed, sleeping all day or taking alcohol or other drugs (Lam et al., 2001).

Through trial and error, many people with bipolar disorder develop a set of personal strategies to manage the depressive side of their illness. We recommend that if a strategy you are already using has been working for you in the long term, treasure it—do not swap it for a newer model. In this and the next few chapters, we present a number of ideas for managing symptoms of depression. The focus of this chapter is on engaging your support network and restoring activity and sleep. You can include any of the ideas you find useful in your plan to prevent or reduce depressive relapse.

THINGS TO KEEP IN MIND

There are a few helpful things to remind yourself about when you notice symptoms of depression:

- **'You are not your depression. You are more than your mood'** (Yapko, 1997:64). Depressed mood can be very real and overwhelming, and feel like a permanent part of your identity, but it is only a mood. Depressive symptoms are part of an illness. Separating yourself from your symptoms can reduce their hold over you and empower you to take action to deal with them. This is often easier the earlier you catch your depression.
- **Depression is not your fault.** 'Depression is not due to an unwillingness to accept responsibility, fears of coping with reality, laziness, cowardice, or weakness' (Miklowitz, 2002:217).
- **There are ways of coping with depressive symptoms.** Feeling anxious if you think you may be developing an episode is not uncommon. Always remember that there are a number of effective treatments and strategies to reduce depression, and that it can be helpful to discuss your worries with someone you trust.

MOBILISING YOUR SUPPORT NETWORK
Contacting your clinician(s)

It is a good idea to contact your doctor for an assessment and to discuss treatment strategies if you think you are becoming depressed. More frequent appointments with your doctor can help you to monitor your depression and put your suicide risk prevention plan into action. Your doctor can arrange hospitalisation if your symptoms are severe or you are in danger of suicide. It can also be useful to contact your psychotherapist or caseworker to assist you with helpful strategies.

Select relatives or friends

Isolating yourself can make you feel more depressed, although many people with bipolar disorder comment that contact with certain individuals can make them feel worse. On the other hand, there may be one or two people who have a positive effect on your mood (Fast & Preston, 2004). In fact, good support has been found to help reduce depressive relapse and the number of days in an episode (Johnson et al., 1999). People with bipolar disorder recommend involving trusted relatives and friends in your plans to stay well (Russell, 2005).

Support from relatives and friends may be practical in the sense of others helping you with actual tasks, and it may also be about experiencing their care and belief in you.

Here are some ideas for ways in which they could be involved:

- finding out about bipolar depression and how you experience it in order to gain more understanding of your situation
- listening to you without judging or criticising you or expecting you to 'snap out of it'
- asking what they can do to help
- supporting your constructive strategies and helping you to reduce stressful triggers and identify and respond to warning symptoms

- helping you monitor your symptoms
- helping out with duties that seem overwhelming but encouraging your efforts to maintain a basic routine or to gradually increase activities
- distracting you by doing things together
- not making too many demands on you and giving you space, but being around
- reassuring you that there are things that help and that, as your symptoms pass, things will look different.

If the depression gets worse, other people can:

- encourage you to call your doctor or call on your behalf
- give you a lift to your clinician or accompany you to the appointment or to hospital if necessary
- help you cancel or delegate commitments if your depression becomes severe or you need to be hospitalised
- help you to use your suicide risk prevention plan (see chapter 13)
- you may instruct them, if it's absolutely necessary, to make urgent treatment decisions on your behalf, and even to discuss what your wishes may be in different circumstances. They need to know that any temporary measures requiring them to step in and act on your behalf are due to the illness and will not be applicable when you are well
- if you are in hospital, visit regularly to show they care
- support your constructive strategies to get back on your feet gradually after an episode of depression, and not to expect too much too soon.

RESTORING ACTIVITY AND SLEEP

Have you noticed how, when you have had a good chat with a friend, enjoyed a funny movie or have managed to achieve something you have been trying to do, things look a bit different? Activities provide experiences that enrich our lives and motivate us. However, when you become depressed it may feel as if doing things and engaging in life is overrated. Even mild symptoms of depression can affect your activity level, enjoyment and motivation.

Going downhill

When you are becoming depressed, things you are usually very capable of doing may become stressful. Sharon, a teacher with bipolar II disorder, began to feel overwhelmed by her everyday routine:

> Demands came at me like tennis balls coming from all directions, and I could not return them. You know when you are playing a game of tennis and you feel hopelessly outmatched? Well, I thought I was just not a good enough player. I rushed around in an anxious frenzy trying to meet demands, but my mind was sluggish and slow. I felt overwhelmed, like I was chasing my tail.

Andrew found that as he became more depressed it was harder to do anything at all, as he felt so lethargic (lacking in energy and tired): 'My body feels heavy and things lose their magic, and in such a dull world all you can do is sleep.'

Going with this lethargy can mean doing less and missing out on the distractions and pleasant experiences that challenge your depressed perspective. Tasks accumulate, making it seem even more overwhelming to do anything. The less you do, the less you feel like doing. This leaves you in a vicious cycle, where you are more vulnerable to typical undermining depressive thinking about how useless you are, which can make you feel even more depressed and less able to do things (see figure 11.1).

Practical activity strategies

Tried and tested psychotherapies (used in conjunction with medication) that reduce depressive relapse in people with

Figure 11.1 The lethargy cycle

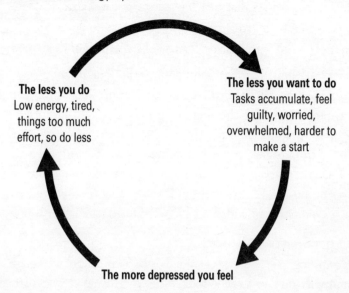

The less you do
Low energy, tired,
things too much
effort, so do less

The less you want to do
Tasks accumulate, feel
guilty, worried,
overwhelmed, harder to
make a start

The more depressed you feel

bipolar disorder include strategies for increasing activities and restoring your usual schedule and sleep habits (Colom et al., 2003a; Lam et al., 2003). Helpful strategies include doing something pleasurable, organising social activity, doing something that provides a sense of mastery or achievement, organising the load, restoring your activity level and building a healthy structure, restoring sleep patterns and getting going in the morning, and exercise.

Do something pleasurable

The experience of pleasure enhances the immune system and improves mood. Fran says: 'Just doing something pleasurable each day, something small for me when I start to notice signs of depression, helps lift me out of the heaviness and makes me a bit more motivated to do other things.' The idea is to create and notice pleasurable experiences. 'By creating even five minutes of amusement, humour, joy, interest, laughter, or pleasure, you are less likely to assume that your negative feelings are chronic and unalterable' (Marra, 2004:149).

If you are not finding much pleasure in things, doing something you used to enjoy may initially provide a sense of satisfaction or achievement and be a distraction. Eventually, as you become more involved in the activity, it may rekindle the old spark of pleasure. It might also be helpful initially to choose activities that do not involve too much effort, like putting on your favourite piece of clothing or spending a few minutes in the garden, then to choose activities that require more planning and input from other people, like going to a movie with friends. A list of ideas for pleasurable activities and a table to assist you in increasing these activities and those that provide a sense of achievement is provided on the website attached to this book.

Organise social activity

Becoming too isolated can enhance depression: although you naturally may feel like withdrawing, socialising can be distracting and enjoyable. You can be selective and choose whose company you would like. Setting small goals to increase your social contact can be a good idea. If you have been cancelling arrangements, you may consider going along for a specified amount of time instead of cancelling. Some people recommend doing an activity with someone else if you find it hard to talk to people, for example, go to a movie or listen to music.

> And in the sweetness of friendship let there be laughter and sharing of pleasures. For in the dew of little things the heart finds its morning and is refreshed.
>
> Khalil Gibran, *The Prophet.*

Do something that provides a sense of mastery or achievement

Experiencing a sense of achievement can be motivating and encourage you to do more. The important thing when you are becoming depressed is to realise that symptoms can get in the way of what you are really capable of doing. For example, you may not be able to concentrate on your work, or have the energy or motivation to perform some task, such as cleaning the house, as you usually do. This is not about your talents or ability but rather what is realistic to expect when you have symptoms of depression. If you have symptoms, it is vital to take your mood into consideration when considering what to expect of yourself. Rani explains, 'Cooking my family a basic meal when I am becoming depressed is as difficult as preparing a fancy cordon bleu dinner party when I am well.'

What will help you to feel a sense of mastery is to know that you have completed something you set out to do, even if it is a step towards a task and not the task itself. The trick is to set goals that are smaller than usual, but still provide a bit of a challenge, and to gradually increase them until you have returned to doing what you usually do.

> I usually love gardening, but when I become depressed I find it hard to do anything so I set myself small tasks. I do a little weeding one day, a little pruning another—the things that don't require much preparation or concentration. Slowly I increase the time and complexity of the tasks and feel pleased with myself if I manage to do them. I know I am improving when I forget to look at my watch, and it no longer feels like such a chore to do what I normally love. **Jim**

Being able to complete a small task before moving on to the next can be a way of both combating lethargy and of getting things done if you experience agitation and restlessness as bipolar symptoms. It really is an achievement to do things when you have symptoms of depression. So acknowledge what you do—for example, reward yourself by relaxing in the garden after working for a half an hour.

Organise the load

Some people initially find organising and planning things for the day or the week 'so boring' or 'an extra chore'; once it's done, however, this can be an effective way of reducing stress, especially if you have symptoms of depression or are recovering from a depressive episode. If your activity level has decreased, or you are feeling overwhelmed and not getting things done, it can be helpful to prioritise what you consider are the most important activities, delegate what you can, and plan a schedule or timetable on a daily or weekly basis. If there are many urgent things to do, consider doing the easiest first. It can be helpful to choose activities that are a bit challenging but not too overwhelming to start with, and then to do more once you achieve them. Assigning a particular time to start an activity can prevent procrastination.

A useful strategy is to break overwhelming tasks down into smaller steps—for example, rather than trying to clean the whole house, decide which room is most urgently in need of attention, and divide that into steps. So, say it's the kitchen, start with the dishes and, once you've done them, go on to the next task, perhaps wiping the benches and then doing the floor. Some people prefer to assign a chunk of time to a task they do not feel like doing. Thus you might decide to spend half an hour cleaning today, and an extra ten minutes tomorrow and 20 minutes the next day. If you are struggling to concentrate on your work, it might be easier to work for half an hour, have a break, then do another half an hour.

Restoring your activity level and building a healthy structure

How many activities you schedule in a day may depend on how depressed you are feeling. If you are battling lethargy, it is important to start small but to see the bigger picture of slowly returning to your usual daily activity schedule. Excessive and frenetic activity to try to catch up with accumulated tasks may result in your feeling very stressed or overstimulated, risking a spiral into an episode of hypomania or mania. Therefore it is very useful to monitor how what you do affects your mood. Rating your mood before and after doing something will inform you about what helps. This way you can control whether you need to introduce more or less or different kinds of activities.

The Mood and Activity Schedule (chapter 16) can help you plan activities that are pleasurable, social and provide a sense of achievement, to organise things and maintain a basic structure. A copy of this schedule is available on www.eburypublishing.co.uk /bipolar.

Do not expect things to change immediately. It takes time to reap the benefits of increasing activity when you have any symptoms of depression. Toby describes his experience: 'I find it hard to get going in the morning and not to sleep in the day, but it is easier since I have things to do and a clear structure to my day.'

Carole, a member of a local bipolar support group, believes in gradually recovering a balanced structure to her week when she feels down: 'I try to get a balance between duties and doing some pleasurable, social and relaxing activities. This means that I don't become too exhausted and stressed out, and still get things done.'

Restoring sleep patterns and getting going in the morning

Depression has a habit of disrupting sleep patterns. Disrupted sleep patterns are both a symptom and an important trigger of bipolar episodes. There are things you can do to help restore this vital aspect of your daily life, such as not sleeping during the day, and there are ways of combating insomnia (see chapter 9). Aim to sleep for eight hours, and schedule a regular activity for when you wake up to help you get out of bed (Colom & Vieta, 2006). When you are increasing and enriching your activities it is important to ensure that they do not disrupt your sleep.

Exercise

Doing exercise when you have any symptoms of depression may seem like trying to defy gravity, develop wings and fly. You may think it is a rude way of waking you from hibernation, but there is growing evidence that exercise helps depression, improves self-esteem and sleep and lowers high anxiety levels (Singh et al., 2001; Spence et al., 2005; Ng et al., 2007). Exercise increases endorphins, the neurotransmitters that improve mood, and reduces stress hormones.

It is important when starting an exercise program to start small and build up gradually. You should first clear this exercise regimen with your doctor, especially if you have major health problems. If you do start to notice symptoms of depression, sticking to your routine exercise program may lessen their severity and hasten your recovery. Taking a friend along to exercise with you can help you to stick to your program.

Doing things with awareness

When you have signs of depression, it is important not only to think of what kind of activities to include in your activity schedule, but also to consider how you do these activities. A common symptom of depression is to be only 'half-present' when you are doing something. Your focus is on your depression and your worries, rather than the task at hand. It is a bit like trying to ride a bike with no hands on the handlebars. Doing things with *awareness* involves a hands-on approach, focusing on what you are doing in the moment (Linehan, 1993). It is putting your attention into the activity itself—for example, if you are making a cup of tea, being aware of the steps involved (choosing a cup, switching on the kettle) and becoming absorbed through your senses in the sights, smells, tastes, touch and sounds involved in doing the activity. You become *involved* in the activity rather than *judging* how you are doing it. If you are anxious about performing a given activity, a good idea is to focus only on the current step, knowing that you can do the same with the next step until the activity is complete.

If self-judgments or any other depressive thoughts and ruminations interrupt your awareness, it helps to simply observe and label them, for example, 'OK, that's critical thinking' or 'worried thinking', and to refocus on the activity itself. Doing things with deliberate awareness may also be useful if you are feeling a bit agitated or restless and flitting from task to task.

When to use activity strategies

Activity strategies need to be used in combination with your other strategies for managing your bipolar disorder. Activity strategies may be easier to use in the early stages of a depressive episode, or when you have warning symptoms or mild ongoing symptoms of depression. Some people find them helpful when trying to combat more severe depression. People have also found them useful when trying to deal with large numbers of accumulated tasks and to regain routines when recovering from an episode of depression.

It is important to keep in mind, however, that if you already feel agitated and overactive due to symptoms of hypomania, mania or mixed states, increasing activities or even exercising may lead to overstimulation and feeling even more hyped up. In these circumstances it may be more helpful to focus on prioritising activities, completing and doing fewer and more relaxing tasks (see chapter 14).

KEY POINTS

- You can do many things to prevent or reduce depressive relapse. Your doctor and other clinicians involved in your treatment, as well as select people in your social network, can be important allies in this regard.

- Activity strategies such as increasing pleasurable activities and those that provide a sense of mastery can help you deal with symptoms of lethargy. Organising the demands and setting small manageable goals to help yourself complete prioritised tasks can make things less overwhelming and stressful. Restoring your routine and sleep habits, exercising, and doing things with awareness can help to stabilise your mood.

- It is always a good idea to use a variety of strategies to tackle depressive symptoms from different angles, including medical treatment and psychotherapy. In the following chapters we look at strategies for reducing pessimistic and undermining thinking and for reducing suicide risk.

12 HELPFUL THINKING STRATEGIES TO REDUCE DEPRESSION

There is nothing either good or bad, but thinking makes it so.
William Shakespeare, *Hamlet*, II, ii, 253

Everyone has some bad days and thinks a bit negatively from time to time. Some people are just prone to seeing the glass as half empty rather than half full, either due to their temperament, or to mild depressive symptoms between episodes of illness. Many people report that their thinking becomes more negative when they are stressed. Instead of being a fleeting negative thought in a difficult situation, this kind of thinking can trigger negative memories and associations about yourself, the world and the future. For some people, negative thinking is a dominant symptom of depression; an increase in negative thinking that is persistent, extreme or rigid is a trusted warning symptom of impending lows. Negative thinking can be very discouraging and immobilising, which leads to your doing less and feeling more depressed. For this reason, it can be helpful to find ways to stop your negative thinking from dragging you down; this chapter suggests some helpful strategies.

DIFFERENT INTERPRETATIONS

There are many different ways of interpreting a situation. Interpretations involve thoughts or 'self-talk' (conversations we all have with ourselves) about the situation. Cognitive behaviourists believe that the way you think about or interpret situations influences your feelings and what you do. For example, if an important meeting at work did not go well you might think: 'I am an idiot, I can't do anything right. I am useless, I might as well resign.' This kind of self-talk may make you feel undermined, angry and sad (feeling) and interfere with your concentration and make it harder to do any work (behaviour). As a result, your work might suffer, which may lead to more negative thinking about how bad you are at your job and make you feel even more distressed.

On the other hand, you might interpret the same situation this way: 'The meeting did not go as well as I hoped and this was due to a number of factors including everyone's lack of preparation. If we take more time to prepare we might improve our chances of selling our product at the next meeting.' You might still feel a bit disappointed, but also empowered to take positive action to deal with the realistic problem.

You can reduce biased, pessimistic and undermining thinking by examining your interpretations and discovering more balanced and helpful perspectives.

UNHELPFUL THINKING STYLES

There are certain typical ways in which your thinking may temporarily become a bit illogical and unhelpful, and thus bias your interpretations of situations, especially when you become depressed or experience mixed states (Basco, 2006). This type of thinking is unhelpful because it can make you feel worse; instead of prompting you to find realistic solutions, if there is a problem, it can immobilise you or result in inappropriate or self-defeating action. Being mindful of these typical thinking distortions can help you to find a more balanced perspective.

They include:

- jumping to negative conclusions
- exaggerating the bad
- extreme thinking.

Jumping to negative conclusions

Jumping to negative conclusions involves judging a situation very quickly and assuming the worst without knowing the full story, or ignoring contradictory evidence. To counteract this tendency, it can be helpful to consider all the evidence before making your judgments. Typical ways of jumping to conclusions include:

Mind-reading

Mind-reading involves jumping to negative conclusions in the belief that you can read a person's mind and know their intentions—for example, 'He thinks I am an idiot', when you don't really know what he thinks. His opinion may be very different from what you imagine it is. Finding out more about what he really thinks may be helpful, and you can remind yourself that no one is a mind-reader.

Personalising

Personalising is taking things personally and jumping to the conclusion that negative things that occur or that someone says are about you, especially when you feel depressed, irritable, suspicious or paranoid. People may have a number of reasons for behaving and responding to you in the way they do—for example, they may be under stress or ill or simply having a bad day. It can be reassuring to consider other possible reasons for another's behaviour—for example, you may assume that 'he is cross with me' when your partner comes home and slams the door. But there may be many other reasons why he slammed the door—work may not have gone as well as he hoped, or he might be feeling very tired or stressed.

Fortune-telling

Fortune-telling involves jumping to conclusions about the future and making negative predictions. It is believing that your guesses about the future are facts. This is common when feeling hopeless or anxious. What helps is to consider other possible outcomes and to realise that you cannot predict the future but you can try to make good things happen—for example, when you have studied hard and there is a good possibility that you will pass, thinking 'I will never pass this test' is fortune-telling.

Blaming

Blaming is the tendency to jump to the conclusion that you or someone else is to blame for something when this is only part of the story or not the case at all. Look for other contributing factors. For example, 'It's my entire fault/your fault that this house is not clean', when there are a number of factors contributing to why the house is not clean.

Mistaking feelings for facts

This is about jumping to the conclusion that because you feel something, it is that way—for example, 'I am scared, it must be dangerous' or 'Because I feel guilty, I am guilty'. Feelings are important but they should not be confused with facts. Feeling something does not make it so; it can be helpful to stand back and make a more objective assessment of the situation.

Exaggerating the bad

When depressed or stressed, you may exaggerate or magnify the negative and bad things that happen and minimise or discount the positive things in yourself, others and the future. Thinking this way can make you feel worse and make it harder to move forward. The important thing here is to look for a more balanced perspective that considers the positives as well. Typical ways in which you may exaggerate the bad include:

Over-generalising

Over-generalising involves reaching sweeping negative conclusions about everything and everyone based on only some of the evidence. You need to remind yourself that only a few pieces of evidence are not the whole story. Other aspects of the situation might contradict your negative view. One bad thing does not mean everyone and everything is bad for all time. It can help to see what went wrong in its specific context. For example, 'I failed this assignment so that means I am useless and might as well give up', may be replaced by 'I failed this assignment but this does not mean I will fail the year, I will find out what went wrong to see how I can do better in the next assignment'.

Catastrophising

Catastrophising is about imagining the worst and blowing things out of proportion. You may exaggerate the consequences or seriousness of a situation or problem, such as failure, rejection or suffering, to a degree with increases your anxiety or hopelessness. A clue to catastrophising is using extreme language to describe consequences, for example, 'terrible', 'disastrous' and 'hopeless'. It can be helpful to look for less drastic possible consequences and to examine whether there is a realistic problem and if so, how it could be solved. For example, the statement 'It is a disaster as I will not be able to find her house' may be substituted with 'It may be a nuisance if I cannot find her house as I may need to ask for directions'. People sometimes underestimate their ability to deal with problems and difficult consequences, and this can make their anxiety worse.

Labelling

Giving negative labels to yourself and others is like putting yourself or them in a box where you will not be able to notice any other qualities or behaviour—for example, 'I am useless'. There is more to a person than a stereotype. Search for a perspective that takes into account different aspects of another person or yourself, and any extenuating circumstances. An alternative response rather than labelling yourself or someone else as 'useless' could be: 'You made a mistake this time but you may do better next time' or 'I'm not good at this particular thing but there are other things that I am good at'.

Extreme thinking

All or nothing thinking

All or nothing thinking involves a tendency to look at things in extreme ways, seeing them as 'very good' or 'terrible' and ignoring the middle ground. Seeking the other side of the story and the grey areas can help. For example, someone you know may have both strengths and flaws.

'Extreme shoulds'

'Extreme shoulds' include the strict rules you may set for yourself, others or life in general, which can become extreme when you feel depressed, such as, 'I should always succeed or I am useless'. Nothing and no one is perfect; we all make mistakes and sometimes unforeseen things happen and situations can be complex. For example, the same person may be understanding or successful in one situation but not in another. There may be many reasons why you or others behave the way you do in particular situations, so dictating how things should always be is not realistic. Having flexible standards that take human fallibility and the complexity of situations into account is more helpful. It is natural to feel disappointed or angry if your expectations are not met but it can be helpful to stand back and examine the 'extreme shoulds' and to see whether you could be less hard on yourself, others and the world. To reduce the pressure of high standards it can be helpful to notice and replace 'I should' or 'I must' with 'I prefer', and to replace 'I have to' with 'I would like' (Tanner & Ball, 1999). For example, 'I would prefer to be a good cook but I am good at other things so it is not a catastrophe if I am not as good at cooking as I would like to be.'

CHALLENGING NEGATIVE OR DEPRESSED THINKING

> Remember that you are not trying to kid yourself that everything is rosy, but you are developing a more balanced perspective on people and events (Tanner & Ball, 1999:70).

In cognitive behavioural therapy, people are assisted to identify, challenge and replace their negative and depressed thinking with more helpful thoughts and actions. Initially this cognitive restructuring is practised on paper until you become used to doing it automatically in your head (Greenberger & Padesky, 1995).

A simple version of this cognitive restructuring technique is the Helpful Thought Summary. The idea is initially to pin down your thinking in specific situations and examine the evidence in those situations to see whether typical unhelpful negative thinking is biasing your interpretation. Then you look for a more balanced interpretation that takes into account the bigger picture and offers a more helpful perspective or way forward, and assess your belief in your original interpretation and how your feelings have changed.

The Helpful Thought Summary

Filling in the Helpful Thought Summary (table 12.1) takes a bit of time at first, but with practice it becomes much easier. To make this easier to understand we present a completed example in table 12.2. There are three main steps involved.

Example using the Helpful Thought Summary

Kathy is a 46-year-old woman with bipolar II disorder who works in advertising. She found the Helpful Thought Summary a convenient way of identifying and challenging her negative thinking in stressful situations and when she was becoming depressed.

She suspected that her thinking in many situations had been particularly negative recently. An example of this was when her

Table 12.1 Helpful thought summary

Step 1: Identify the situation, negative thoughts and do ratings
If you know that your thinking has been rather negative lately, you may be able to catch specific negative thoughts by examining your thinking in specific situations.

1. Situation
Think of a recent situation and write down what happened. Stick to the facts and give details to prevent the chance of misinterpretation.

2. Thought
Try to remember some of the thoughts that were going through your head in the situation. You may have a number of thoughts. Choose the one that is most intense or prominent to work on first. The acronym SOB sums up some of the negative thinking that sometimes occurs automatically and may stimulate your memory:

S: Self-critical
- Did you experience critical, undermining, blaming thoughts about yourself in the situation?

O: Others' opinions or opinions about the world
- Did you think that others were critical, hostile or rejecting towards you in that situation?
- Did you have critical, suspicious or hostile thoughts about others in that situation?

B: Bad future
- Did you experience pessimistic, hopeless, worried or suicidal thoughts?
- You may find a number of negative thoughts and you can choose to challenge the most intense or 'hot' thought and then to go on to challenge the others.

continued

3. Rate
- How much you *believe* the thought as a percentage between 0 and 100 per cent.
- How you *felt* in the situation or how the thought makes you feel, for example, sad, anxious, and angry as a percentage between 0 and 100 per cent.

These ratings will be useful to use when reviewing how your belief and feelings change once you have challenged your thinking.

Step 2: Challenge unhelpful negative thinking
Once you have identified the negative thinking you can challenge it by looking at it from different perspectives (Edelman, 2002).

1. Separate the facts of the situation from your opinion or interpretation.
Be mindful not to confuse fact and opinion. Facts refer to actual events, actions or conversation. We may have different explanations and opinions about these facts. Also, remember that feeling something does not make it a fact—for example, you may feel rejected but this does not mean that you are rejected. We sometimes can interpret rejection when it is not there.

2. List evidence for and against your interpretation
The following questions may help with this:
What evidence supports my thought or interpretation?
What evidence is there that brings my interpretation into question?
For example:
- What other interpretations of the situation are there?
- Are there other possible contributing factors that I am not recognising?
- Is there other evidence that I am ignoring that supports a different interpretation to mine?

continued

- If someone else were in this situation, what would I say to help them interpret this situation in a balanced way?
- How would a good friend or someone I trust see the situation?
- Am I seeing things in a biased way and using any of the unhelpful thinking styles mentioned above?

Step 3: Helpful response; re-rating your belief and feeling
The next step is to find and act on a more balanced perspective.

1. What is an alternative, more logical and helpful perspective in the long term?

Write down a more helpful thought that takes the evidence and different interpretations into account. There may be more than one helpful alternative thought.

2. What positive action(s) can you take in response to your new interpretation?

Usually this process will broaden your perspective on the situation and it becomes possible to see a specific action that can help you move forward.

3. Rate how strongly you now believe your negative thought and the intensity of your feelings in the situation that you identified previously (0 to 100 per cent).

See if this has altered from your ratings when you started this exercise.

friend Pete, was not very talkative at a dinner arrangement the previous evening, and left early. She interpreted this to mean that he wanted to end their relationship.

Kathy examined her thinking using the three steps described in table 12.1. When she had done so (see table 12.2), Kathy felt a little better and called Pete. She discovered that he was very stressed about his move to a new house, and was pleased to have her offer of support. This confirmed her more balanced perspective.

Table 12.2 Kathy's helpful thought summary

1. Identify	2. Challenge	3. Helpful response
Situation	**Facts and opinions**	**Helpful thought**
Went out for dinner together. Pete spoke very little and left to go home at 9 pm.	The facts are that he did speak less than usual and he left early, but it is my opinion that the reason for this is that he wanted to end the relationship.	That Pete wanted to end the friendship is a possible explanation, but his behaviour in the past contradicts this. There may be other explanations connected to his current situation.
Thought	**Evidence for**	
He wants to end the relationship.	He left early and was not as talkative as usual.	
Rate belief and feelings	**Evidence against**	**Helpful action**
Unhelpful thought 95% Sad at loss 90% Anxious about friendship 95%	He also gets depressed and may be feeling down. He is moving house this week and may be worried about it or need to pack. Pete has told me previously that he enjoys my company, and nothing has happened between us since I last saw him to explain why he would want to end the friendship. I may be mind-reading, fortune-telling, personalising things, exaggerating the bad and using 'extreme shoulds'.	Perhaps I will give him a call ask him if he is OK or upset with me as I noticed he was quieter than usual and left early. I can also offer to help with the move if that is making him feel stressed.
		Re-rate beliefs and feelings
		Unhelpful thought 40% Sad 40% Anxious 50%

Underlying patterns

Kathy realised that when she felt stressed or depressed, she frequently jumped to the conclusion that people were rejecting her. Another pattern she noticed was that she tended to blame herself excessively when things did not happen as planned at work, instead of looking at all the factors that may have contributed to the situation. As Kathy explains:

Negative thinking has been a strong early symptom of depression for me, and standing back and observing my thinking, rather than being drawn in by it, made me realise something astonishing. I noticed that there were patterns in my unhelpful thinking.

While I am usually achievement driven, and am quite sensitive in my interpersonal relationships, when I am becoming depressed, this pattern of negative thinking becomes extreme and I interpret every little thing at work as confirmation that I am an idiot and in my personal relationships as rejection. I called these my 'I am an idiot thoughts' [S: self-critical thoughts] and 'Everyone is rejecting me thoughts' [O: others' opinions] as this made them easy to identify. If these go on, I get the 'I have no future thoughts' [B: bad future]. Since it has become easier to identify my negative thinking, it has less power over me, and I can distance myself from it and more easily replace it with a more balanced perspective.

Have a go yourself

You will find a copy of the Helpful Thought Summary on the website associated with this book. You can use it to challenge and replace your negative thinking. Sometimes you may need to repeat this process a number of times and challenge other thoughts that are connected to your depressed feeling before you notice a change. Although this process may seem lengthy at first, with practice it becomes easier and enables you to identify unhelpful patterns of thinking and helpful responses. Some people find it useful to keep a short list of their typical negative thinking patterns and helpful responses to use when necessary. You can draw up such a list on the website attached to this book.

EXTRA TIPS
Test your helpful response

Think of practical ways that you can test your negative thinking and confirm your helpful response in real life. This can provide useful evidence when challenging similar future negative thinking. Kathy in the example above could remind herself that last time she jumped to the conclusion that someone was rejecting her, other possible explanations were confirmed by her helpful action of checking this out. She could use this as future evidence.

Realistic problems and goals

Sometimes in the process of challenging negative thinking, you may uncover realistic problems. Problem solving is a useful technique for dealing with the problems that are revealed by challenging your negative thinking (see chapter 19 and the website associated with this book). It is sometimes harder to find solutions when you are depressed, as negative thinking may make you catastrophise the problem, anticipate the worst and underestimate your ability to deal with the problem. It might be an idea to address your negative thinking first, so it does not get in the way of solving the problem. Enlisting the support of a trusted friend or clinician in problem solving can make a difference. Viewing the problem as a goal can help (Scott, 2001). For example, instead of worrying about a problem with your partner, it may be helpful to view improving communication as a goal and plan the first step, such as arranging a time to discuss things.

Underlying negative assumptions

You may find that there are unrealistic 'core beliefs' underneath the automatic way you interpret and think about situations when your mood is low, such as 'I have to be good at everything or no one will like me' (Greenberger & Padesky, 1995). Finding evidence that contradicts these beliefs can make it easier to reduce your negative thinking. In order to get to this underlying belief you can ask yourself, 'If this negative thought I am having were true, what would it mean to me?' You will probably come up with another automatic thought, if you keep asking the question you may get to your underlying belief. Trained cognitive behavioural therapists can be helpful in picking up and challenging negative thinking and underlying beliefs.

For more detailed information on tackling negative thinking we recommend Basco's *Bipolar Workbook* (2006), *Mind over Mood* by Greenberger & Padesky (1995) and Edelman's *Change Your Thinking* (2002).

REPETITIVE AND PERSISTENT NEGATIVE THINKING

Depressed thinking can become so repetitive and persistent that it is hard to think of other things; we refer to this phenomenon as *rumination*. Besides the cognitive reconstruction techniques discussed above and the medications you take to stabilise your mood, other strategies have been recommended to reduce intense negative thinking, including changing your relationship with your thinking, distraction, saying 'Stop', and making a special 'worry time'.

Change your relationship with your depressed thinking

> It is remarkable how liberating it feels to be able to see that your thoughts are just thoughts and that they are not 'you' or 'reality' (Kabat-Zinn, 1990:67).

Distancing yourself from your depressed thinking can make it less threatening and reduce its hold over you. This does not mean trying not to think negatively. Rather, it is about letting the negative thoughts appear but seeing that they are just thoughts and neutralising their negative effect.

People might think that frogs live on the moon, but that is just a thought. Kathy, in the example above, was able to identify her depressed thought patterns and recognise that they were only opinions, heavily influenced by her growing negative mood. She did not have to believe or act on them. She realised that she was more than her thoughts or even her mood. She looked 'at' her negative thinking rather than viewing the world 'from' it. This altered her relationship to her thinking.

There are strategies people can use so they do not 'fuse' or 'buy' into their negative thoughts (Hayes & Smith, 2005). Rather than changing the content of your thinking, Mindfulness-Based Cognitive Therapy (Segal et al., 2002) teaches you mindfulness meditation techniques. These get you used to standing back and observing your feelings, bodily sensations and thoughts without being drawn in by them. The usefulness of these approaches for people with bipolar disorder is currently being studied.

Distraction

Doing something pleasurable, or even a chore, can be distracting as long as it means that you are focused on something else. Involving yourself in an activity may help you to be absorbed in the outside world rather than focused in your head. Some people find that imagining a pleasurable or calming experience helps to interrupt the rumination.

Having a pleasurable experience or gaining a sense of mastery from what you are doing can make you feel more positive when the distracting activity ends, which also makes it easier to distance yourself from ruminative thoughts.

Saying 'stop'

Some people find it useful to say 'stop', either aloud or in their mind, or clap their hands when ruminating, then shift to doing something distracting.

A special worry time

Another strategy is scheduling a specific worrying or ruminating time each day, with a specific time limit that involves something you have to do, say going to eat dinner when the half hour is up.

MORE ABOUT MANAGING WORRIES

Some people with bipolar disorder spend a lot of time worrying. A little bit of anxiety may be helpful when it gives you a message to prepare well for a particular event, but constant worry may do the opposite. Lots of worry can be unhelpful, not only because it interferes with your concentration and therefore can jeopardise your performance, but also because it makes you feel vulnerable and unsafe and can lead to avoidance of fulfilling activities—for example, not undertaking a course of study because you want to avoid the anxiety about taking the exam. Worry can do the opposite of what you expect. Rather than helping you to cope better with life, it can impair your ability to function properly, and this may add to your stress and negative thinking.

I think I believed in some strange way that worrying about something would help me to control it. I would not be taken unawares. I did a little experiment and examined the outcome of things I worried about and things I didn't. As a result, I realised that whether or not I worried made little difference to how things turned out. In fact, sometimes my worry made me freeze up so that I couldn't do anything. Then I just avoided everything and became more depressed. I noticed that what did help was to work out ways of tackling things step by step and having a plan A and B. I also realised that there are ways of surviving and coping when things do not go according to plan B. My life became less restricted as I stopped worrying so much and avoiding things. **Frank**

There are alternative ways of dealing with difficult situations besides worrying or avoiding them. We mention a few tips below, including challenging anxious thinking, preparing yourself with effective coping skills, and reversing bodily changes. For more detail on ways of reducing worry and anxiety disorders, we refer you to the helpful resources listed on the website associated with this book. You may also benefit from engaging in psychotherapy to help you find suitable strategies to manage your anxiety.

Challenging anxious thinking

Challenging your anxious thinking about a situation and replacing it with a more balanced assessment can reduce catastrophising, predicting the worst and underestimating your ability to cope, which are all part of anxious thinking. Accepting that things not working out the way you plan is part of life, and that it is usually possible to deal with even the worst possible consequences and still survive, can relieve worry. Anticipation is very often much worse than the reality; finding concrete examples of this that have occurred in your life can be reassuring.

Preparing yourself with effective coping skills

You can prepare yourself for a situation by assessing what is required, and learning and rehearsing coping skills so you can put them into practice in that situation. For example, if you have an exam or important meeting you could prepare yourself and in your mind's eye imagine handling different aspects. Anticipating difficulties does not mean you have to worry about them. Working out possible solutions beforehand equips you to manage if things go wrong.

Reversing physical changes

Techniques that target the physical changes that occur when we experience anxiety, such as relaxation techniques, may help to calm you (see chapter 18).

WHEN TO CHALLENGE NEGATIVE THINKING

Negative thinking styles may make you more vulnerable to relapse when stressors occur. Some people find that challenging their negative thinking when they are in a stressful situation prevents such thinking from getting worse. Consciously trying to maintain a balanced perspective can be part of a healthy lifestyle. These techniques may also be beneficial if you have residual symptoms between episodes, when you notice warning or early symptoms of depression and during an episode of depression, together with other strategies for managing your illness. The less entrenched the depressive thinking, the easier it is to challenge.

KEY POINTS

- The aim is not to abolish all negative thinking. Everyone thinks negatively and worries from time to time. When these thoughts are not just occasional and fleeting, they can contribute to your swing into depression. It can be useful to try to maintain a balanced perspective as part of a healthy lifestyle and to challenge negative thinking under times of stress in order to prevent stressors from triggering depression.
- In this chapter we have discussed ways of managing unhelpful negative thinking, including repeatedly challenging and replacing it with more helpful alternatives, detecting patterns so that you can respond to this symptom as early as possible, and a few strategies for reducing rumination and worry.
- Helpful thinking strategies should be used in conjunction with the other strategies, and together they may help you to prevent or reduce relapse.

- These strategies need practice, and there are resources to make this easier.
- Enlisting the help of a cognitive therapist can assist you in reducing negative thinking and worry.

13 REDUCING SUICIDE RISK

While you are waiting for the crisis to subside, be patient.
This will pass, but only if you stay alive.

Madeleine Kelly, *Life on a Roller Coaster*, 2000:133.

Thoughts about ending one's life are experienced by many, but not all people with bipolar disorder. The most common time for feeling suicidal, and the period of highest risk for suicide attempts is *during* or just *after* a depressive or mixed episode, although some people have suicidal thoughts between episodes of illness. People who experience a dysphoric type of mania may feel suicidal.

Suicidal thoughts or impulses should always be taken seriously. People with bipolar disorder are 15 times more likely to die from suicide than people who do not have the illness (Harris & Barraclough, 1997). Certain risk factors can alert you and others to be extra vigilant in dealing with your suicide risk; these include a previous suicide attempt, being isolated from others, having recently experienced a major stressful event, feeling hopeless or already having a plan to commit suicide, abusing drugs or alcohol or having an anxiety disorder (Rihmer, 2007).

The good news is that you and those around you can do a lot to reduce the risk and to prevent suicide, and we outline some possibilities in this chapter. No one likes dwelling on suicidality, but examining helpful ways of coping with this distressing and all-too-common symptom may prove an advantage if it arises. We discuss identifying suicide risk and developing a personal prevention plan that you can use when you are ill.

SIGNS OF SUICIDE RISK

Sometimes people have early warnings of impending suicidality which can alert them to take action. Thoughts that life is not worthwhile, for example, might precede thoughts of actual self-harm. At other times, actual suicidal thoughts and impulses can raise the alarm.

Warning signs might include specific triggers and mood symptoms, or red-alert signals of immediate danger. No matter when you identify suicide risk, there are things you can do to prevent suicide. Picking up early signs can make this easier.

Triggers

Some people find that specific triggers, for example, conflict in a valued relationship or a negative event such as the end of a relationship, social isolation, pressure at work, or too much alcohol or drugs, especially when combined with bipolar moods, can lead them to consider suicide. Finding different ways of dealing with these particular problems, and getting well, may reduce these suicidal feelings.

Other symptoms

Some people have warning signs which are also typical bipolar symptoms, such as hopelessness, withdrawal, agitation, or an increase in anxiety or guilt. They may be similar to your warning signs of depressive or mixed episodes. If you know that when you experience these warning symptoms you tend to become suicidal, you can take action to reduce your suicide risk early, before the impulse becomes very severe, by putting your action plan to prevent suicide risk into practice, together with your other strategies to manage your illness.

It is particularly useful to catch hopelessness early. Acknowledging and sharing your hopelessness and challenging the one-sided thinking connected to this feeling can help to prevent hopelessness from becoming too overwhelming. Viewing your hopelessness as a temporary symptom rather than a true reflection of reality makes it easier to commit to not performing any self-defeating action, such as resigning, ending a relationship or planning suicide.

It is vital to look out for hopelessness not only as an early warning of suicidal impulses but also as a danger sign once an episode is over. In the aftermath of an episode, with all the pressures that descend on you, hopelessness sometimes persists even when your other symptoms subside. The risk of suicide may increase as your energy returns. For this reason, it is important to give yourself enough time to get through this vulnerable period, even though you feel much better, to lessen the risk of acting on your hopelessness. In time, once you are fully recovered, you are likely to see things very differently. Your difficulties and problems may not have disappeared, but what changes is that you can find more solutions and aspects of life that you enjoy and value.

Danger signs

Thinking about suicide is an important symptom to communicate to others. Other signs to look out for include starting to give things away, resigning from commitments, writing letters to deal with unfinished business, and fixing up your will. If such signs that you are feeling suicidal or even planning a suicide attempt appear, you need to take immediate action to reduce the risk. Having a plan to commit suicide is a red-alert signal of impending danger and you need urgent help. If you have attempted suicide before, your risk is increased.

AN ACTION PLAN TO PREVENT SUICIDE

Sometimes when you are suicidal the experience feels all too real, and it is hard to see it as a temporary symptom of illness, and recognise that there are other ways of finding relief from your distress. For this reason, it is a good idea to plan strategies for managing suicide risk when you are well. Your suicide risk prevention plan can then be put into practice as soon as you start to feel suicidal or notice warning signs of impending suicidality. In order to draw up such a plan, you will need to consider what you and those close to you can do to reduce your risk of suicide. Some ideas for taking action to prevent suicide are presented below.

What can you do?

Your safety is a priority if you are feeling suicidal. Remember, there are things you can do to stay safe and get help. You can also do things that will help you get through this time and reduce your suicidal thoughts and other mood symptoms.

Safety first

- Phone your clinician and let them know about your suicidal thoughts or plans, and book an emergency appointment.
- Call your local hospital emergency department if you cannot contact your usual clinician.
- Remove access to medications, pills, car keys or anything else that you could use to harm yourself.
- Let key family and friends know that you are feeling suicidal.
- Stay with someone so that you are not alone.

- If your suicidal thoughts increase or you develop a plan to suicide, or if you or others consider you are in imminent danger, call your doctor again or go to an emergency department.
- Drugs and alcohol can make your mood worse and lead to impulsive acts, so it is vital to abstain from these if you are feeling suicidal.

Getting through this time

- Talk things through with a trusted person or call a suicide hotline.
- Get some distance from your suicidal thoughts by recognising that they are only temporary symptoms and that you do not have to agree with them or act on them.
- Just focus on getting through the next hour of the day. When you are very ill, breaking time into manageable bits is easier than considering getting through the future.
- What can help you get through the moment is to do things that make your distress easier to tolerate and that could lift your mood. Examples include spending time with a loved one; doing something that is soothing, such as listening to music; expressing your feelings through art, writing or playing a musical instrument; praying; playing with a pet and doing relaxation exercises (Linehan, 1993).
- Do things such as going to the mall, a park, the library or the movies that distract you from your suicidal thoughts.
- If religion or spirituality is meaningful to you, you could consider seeking support from religious or spiritual leaders or friends who share your beliefs.

Reducing symptoms

- Put your strategies for reducing relapse into practice and discuss treatment with your doctor. Some medications can decrease the agitation, anxiety and impulsiveness that can drive suicidal impulses.
- Identify your negative thinking and find more helpful perspectives. The fact that you are temporarily feeling hopeless *does*

not mean that things are hopeless. You may feel very differently about things in the future.

- Often suicide is not about wanting to die but about wanting to escape situations or problems in which you feel hopeless and stuck. Finding new solutions or new ways of responding to old problems can make you feel very differently about the future and reduce your hopelessness. It can be helpful to brainstorm alternative ways of dealing with old problems and situations with a clinician or a trusted friend or relative.
- Prioritise and delegate stressful demands that make you feel overwhelmed.
- Ask yourself what might make a difference in the future so you have something to work towards (Miklowitz, 2002). For example, 'It would make a difference if my illness was under control', '. . . if I had a relationship' or '. . . if I find something I want to do'. Then decide to work towards this objective and to get well in the meantime.

Compile a Reasons to Live List

Often, when we ask people with a previous history of suicide attempts whether they feel suicidal, they say that occasionally they still think of suicide but not seriously, because they have thought of reasons to live. You could develop a Reasons to Live List when you are well (see www.eburypublishing.co.uk/bipolar) and keep it in easy reach for the times when you feel suicidal. The list does not need to contain many items, as long as they are meaningful to you (Linehan et al., 1983, Miklowitz, 2002).

Examples include:

- You don't want to devastate your children, family or friends.
- You want to watch your children grow up.
- You can't leave those you love.
- You have a responsibility towards those you love.
- Things might be different in the future.

- You can make things different in the future and learn to adjust to your problems.
- There are still things you want to experience and things you want to do.
- Your suicidal feelings are temporary symptoms of illness, and you cannot let them control your life
- When you are well, there are things that mean a lot to you.
- You are scared that your suicide attempt will fail and you will be left damaged in some way.
- You believe it is morally or religiously wrong to commit suicide.
- You are not sure what happens when you die.
- You have a mission or purpose in life.
- You are concerned about what other people will think.
- There is hope that things will improve.

What can others do to help?

Although suicidality is a dangerous symptom of illness, it is unfortunately often a taboo topic. A recent survey found that out of 69 per cent of people with bipolar disorder who had suicidal thoughts, only 49 per cent discussed these thoughts with their doctor (Lewis & Hoofnagle, 2005). Suicidal impulses can be managed and controlled, and it is important not to feel alone with or to be ashamed of this common symptom of bipolar disorder. Some people are reluctant to tell their doctor, their psychologist or a close family member or friend about their hopelessness or suicidal thoughts, because they think the other person will not be able to help. Yet in reality there is a lot they can do to help (Miklowitz, 2002).

What your clinician can do

Your doctor can listen to you, assess the severity of your suicide risk, review your medications, and recommend appropriate treatment and ways of keeping safe until your mood lifts. This may involve seeing you more often to help you monitor your suicidal thoughts and other symptoms, suggesting alternative ways of dealing with your distress and the factors that contribute to it, and organising hospitalisation if necessary. Added support from a psychologist, combined with your own strategies to relieve your distress and prevent suicide, can make things easier.

How family and friends can help

Not everyone has close family members or friends whom they can call on if they feel suicidal. When you do have such people, they can be valuable allies. Sometimes they too feel helpless, being unsure of what to do when you are suicidal. It can be useful to discuss ways they could be supportive that might suit both of you and which you can include in your plan to reduce suicide risk. Ways in which they might boost your constructive coping strategies include:

- Taking away weapons, medications or anything else you think may be potentially lethal and storing them for you temporarily and discussing how they can help you to feel more safe.
- Spending time with you until your suicidal impulses pass.
- Really listening to you and trying to understand your feelings, without being critical.
- Brainstorming with you to find alternative solutions to difficulties that seem overwhelming and to create new achievable goals that make you feel more hopeful about the future.
- Temporarily helping out with burdensome demands, such as childcare.
- Reminding you that these suicidal feelings are temporary and you may see things quite differently in the future.
- Distracting you through doing pleasant things together, such as going for a drive or watching a movie.
- Calling your doctor or the hospital emergency department on your behalf if necessary, and driving you there.
- Acting in your best interest even if you are temporarily so ill that you cannot see alternatives.

DEVELOPING YOUR SUICIDE RISK PREVENTION PLAN

You can review the suggestions above and add your own ideas to develop your personal Suicide Risk Prevention Plan. There is a template for you to use on the website associated with this book. The idea of a Suicide Risk Prevention Plan is to compile contact numbers of people who have agreed to help if you become suicidal, and a list of very specific things that you and others have agreed to do to prevent suicide and help you through this time. If it's possible, it is a good idea to have a few other people you trust involved in your plan in the event that your key person is away. Remember the option of contacting the hospital emergency department if your clinician is not available. Keep the instructions simple and brief so that the plan is easy to use when you are ill. The next thing is to give everyone involved a copy of your list so that they have it to hand if the need arises. Some people like getting everyone involved to sign and keep a copy of the plan so that it becomes a contract. Contracts are meant to be honoured.

Another tip is to put your plan into action as early as possible, as it can be more difficult once your symptoms become severe. Also, remember to update your plan as circumstances change (especially new names and phone numbers) and when you have new ideas.

Figure 13.1, Jane's Suicide Risk Prevention Plan, is a worked example. You may find that you have different strategies, and we emphasise the need to personalise your plan according to what works for you.

Jane had suffered from bipolar disorder for three years and found that when she became severely depressed she tended to become suicidal. She had previously attempted suicide and was very relieved to be alive. She was worried that this might happen again so she decided to take control of things and reduce this risk.

Her Suicide Risk Prevention Plan involves things she can do, and the help of her husband Jeff, her sister Caron and her parents, as well as her clinicians.

Figure 13.1 Jane's suicide risk prevention plan

Contact details

Doctors' names and phone numbers:

Dr Patterson (psychiatrist): 9453 5487 or 9457 7777

Dr Leeb (GP): 9498 7652 or 0467 544 111

Psychologist/case worker's name and phone number

Cindy Tong 9457 3888

Emergency Dept phone number: 1432

Close family or friends

Jeff at work: 9457 6891 or 0423 786 454

Caron at work: 9457 8690 or home: 9465 7687 or 0478 453 766

Parents: 0485 567 078 or 9456 9084

Early warning signs that I may become suicidal

(List warning signs that you may be becoming suicidal if you have experienced any. These may be similar to your early symptoms of depression or mixed states or be specific to becoming suicidal.)

Look out for:

- hopelessness
- cancelling arrangements and wanting to resign
- crying a lot

What I can do about warning signs

(List ways of dealing with your warning signs)

- Activate my action plan to manage symptoms of depression and Suicide Risk Prevention Plan.
- Challenge early hopeless thinking and problem solve if there is a specific problem that may be triggering my hopelessness, together with Cindy.

continued

- Make no decisions about resigning.
- Monitor my hopelessness and do pleasant distracting things. If it persists, gets worse or I become suicidal call Dr Patterson.

Consider safety and getting treatment
(What do you need to do to ensure your safety and access to treatment?)
- Contact Dr Patterson or Dr Leeb, discuss symptoms, and arrange emergency appointment for assessment and to discuss best treatment.
- Keep Jeff, my parents and Caron up to date about my symptoms so they can help monitor my suicidality
- Give all my pills to Jeff temporarily and let him lock away the medicines and his gun.
- Try not to be alone. Be with parents if Jeff at work.
- Monitor my symptoms and suicidal thoughts, and if they get worse or I start thinking of a plan to commit suicide communicate this to my family and call (family may need to call) the doctor and go to hospital.

Other strategies I can use and ways others can assist me
(What other strategies can make things easier and reduce your suicidality?)
- Schedule more frequent appointments with my doctor and psychologist and discuss other ways of coping with my distress and lifting my mood.
- Distract myself from suicidal thoughts by watching TV, painting, and doing gardening, and put my relapse prevention plan for depression into practice.
- Spend time with the people I care about and do distracting things together, for example, shopping, art galleries, go for drives (Caron, Jeff, parents).
- Keep my Reasons to Live List in easy reach and remind myself about what is important to me when I feel well.
- Challenge my negative thinking distortions, like exaggerating the bad and predicting the future, using the Helpful Thought

continued

Summary. Tell myself that feeling suicidal and having suicidal thoughts does not mean that I have to act on them and that they will pass as they have before.

- Reduce stressful demands: try to extend the deadlines on my part-time contract work or subcontract the work and arrange for Jeff, Caron and my parents to take over some of my chores, temporarily.

- Use the Mood and Activity Schedule to make sure I maintain some activities and try to do pleasurable things. Cindy, my psychologist, can help with this.

Signatures: . . . .

KEY POINTS

- Suicide is a serious risk in bipolar disorder, but there is a lot you can do to reduce your personal risk.
- Catching triggers and warning signs of suicidality can alert you and others to take action and reduce the risk. Hopelessness and signs of suicidality need to be taken seriously.
- Safety is always the first priority. There are strategies for managing your current mood and helping you get through this time, and there are alternative ways of sorting out problems. Drawing up a Reasons to Live List to use at these times is also helpful.
- Feeling suicidal is a heavy and potentially dangerous burden to deal with all alone, and there is a lot both your clinicians and other key people in your life can do to lessen the burden and reduce the risk. Dealing with this serious aspect of your bipolar disorder as a team can make a difference.
- Developing your own Suicide Risk Prevention Plan together with these key people provides direction and safety at high-risk times.

14

MANAGING WARNING SYMPTOMS OF HYPOMANIA OR MANIA

Recognising that you have warning signs of any illness can be a bit scary, but I have learnt to monitor them and call my doctor. The medication my doctor prescribes when I am becoming manic helps me sleep, and I take frequent special quiet times when I stand back and slow down. This gives me more control, and I can prevent a full relapse.
Julie

When you notice warning symptoms of mania or hypomania, there are things that you can do to prevent full relapse. People who respond to their warning signs by using constructive behavioural strategies, such as consulting their doctor, spending quiet time resting, doing calming things, and reducing extreme behaviour and unhelpful thinking have fewer relapses and enjoy better functioning in their relationships and working lives than those who engage in unhelpful ways of coping (Lam et al., 2001). Unhelpful ways of coping include increasing your level of stimulation, spending more money, and ignoring your warning signs.

Your plans to prevent or reduce hypomanic or manic relapse can include a few key personally relevant warning signs, and basic instructions about what to do and what not to do, so that you can respond early, constructively and quickly. In this chapter we focus on consulting your doctor, strategies for reducing overactivity and restoring sleep, and dealing with early changes in thinking in order to catch early symptoms and prevent relapse. The next chapter suggests ways of preventing some of the unfortunate consequences sometimes connected with mania.

THINGS TO KEEP IN MIND

Timing is important when you want to prevent an episode. The problem with the trip up the roller-coaster is that many people do not know when they are reaching the top. As they become more hypomanic or manic, their insight into the fact that they are ill can diminish, so that they see less point in taking medications or using helpful strategies to control their symptoms. Picking up warning symptoms early and responding promptly can make a difference.

While you are still separate from your illness, you have the opportunity to control how you want to respond. You can try to hold on to the idea that your feelings and ideas are temporarily influenced by your growing hypomanic mood and that you do not have to act on them. This gives you a chance to put your relapse prevention strategies into practice. Separating yourself from your illness can help you and those around you to put your symptomatic behaviour into perspective and reduce the blame, guilt and disruption to your life.

Many people recognise that they cycle from hypomania or mania into depression and so, even if their hypomania or mania is pleasant, they act promptly to reduce it in order to prevent the swing into depression. Others are determined to take action to prevent or reduce mania due to the risk of negative consequences and the disruption it can cause. Many people are encouraged by the knowledge that there are effective ways of preventing and reducing relapse.

EARLY TREATMENT

People with bipolar disorder who identify warning signs of illness and contact their doctor in order to get help can nip a hypomanic or manic episode in the bud by taking appropriate prescribed medication before it develops into a full relapse (Perry et al., 1999). Regular contact with your doctor and follow-up is also helpful (Simon et al., 2006). Your doctor can assess your mood and organise hospitalisation on your behalf if things get worse.

If you and your doctor have worked together for some time, and you are experienced at recognising your warning signs, your doctor may organise with you when you are well to take additional prescribed medication to slow down and restore sleep when you notice warning signs of episodes. The idea is to keep monitoring your warning signs and let your doctor know if your mood does not improve or gets worse. You may need to request that your doctor see you earlier than your next scheduled appointment if things are not improving. Catching your manic symptoms early might reduce the chance of ending up in hospital. Some people have other clinicians, such as a psychologist or a case manager, involved in their treatment, and it may be helpful to contact them as well to bolster your strategies to prevent relapse.

SLOW DOWN AND GET SOME SLEEP

Studies have shown that when you have bipolar disorder, disruption to regular activities, social stimulation and sleep patterns can upset your body clock or circadian rhythms and trigger hypomania or mania (Frank, 2007). When you are becoming hypomanic or manic, you may feel as if you have suddenly gone into the fast lane and have loads of ideas, your activity level speeds up and you sleep less. This disruption in turn can make you spin deeper and deeper into an episode of illness. You can use a number of strategies in addition to taking prescribed medication to interrupt this activity cycle and restore your body clock.

The activity cycle

In depression, all aspects of mood, including biology, behaviour, thoughts and feelings, reinforce each other as you sink deeper into depression in a downward spiral. In the lethargy cycle, the less you do, the less you want to do, as your depression gets worse. In mania we see the opposite occur as an activity cycle spins you deeper into that state (see figure 14.1). Doing lots of activities makes you feel energised and overstimulated, making things speed up so that you think, move and do more, disrupting your usual

Figure 14.1 The activity cycle

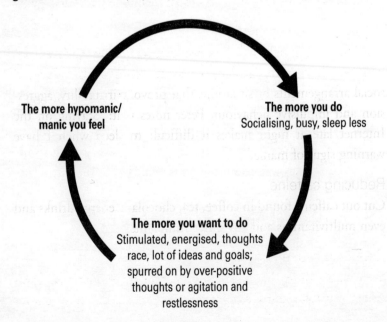

The more hypomanic/
manic you feel

The more you do
Socialising, busy, sleep less

The more you want to do
Stimulated, energised, thoughts
race, lot of ideas and goals;
spurred on by over-positive
thoughts or agitation and
restlessness

routine and sleep patterns. The more you do, the more you want to do. The activity cycle has its own momentum and it may be spurred on by increasingly optimistic and confident thoughts. This means that strategies to help you slow down, restore your regular activity, level of stimulation and sleep habits may be helpful. You need to start putting the brakes on early.

Putting the brakes on

People with bipolar disorder recommend a number of strategies to reduce stimulation, restore routines, and sleep patterns.

Getting more sleep

Getting too little sleep is a major trigger of hypomania and mania, and many people report that regulating their sleep restores stability. Some experts recommend increasing your sleep to at least 10 hours with the temporary assistance of medication prescribed by your doctor (Colom & Vieta, 2006). They suggest that as an emergency plan, sleeping a lot for a few days may be sufficient to ward off an episode of hypomania or mania. You could also try the additional strategies for restoring your sleep mentioned in chapter 9.

Reducing overstimulation

Consider what is personally overstimulating for you. For example, while you have warning signs, stay away from crowds and lots of social arrangements or situations that provoke irritability, aggression and impulsive behaviour. Peter notes that: 'Staying on the Internet late at night makes it difficult to sleep when I have warning signs of mania.'

Reducing caffeine

Cut out caffeine found in coffee, tea, chocolate, energy drinks and even multivitamins and any other stimulants.

Reducing causes of aggravation

See whether things happening around you are temporarily aggravating your symptoms, such as loud TV, music, children's clutter or lots of entertaining. Enlisting the support of your household makes reducing such stimulation a shared task.

Choosing calming activities

If you are struggling with lots of pent-up energy and difficulty in sitting still, choose the activity that is least stimulating. For example, if you feel like going for a 10 kilometre run and know you will feel even more hyped up afterwards, choose a gentler walk around the block, or go for a drive with a good friend rather than to a party. Do not try to exhaust yourself by doing much more exercise and activity as this will just make you more stimulated and make you more hypomanic or manic.

Reducing numbers of activities

Reduce overactivity by planning fewer activities for the week. 'You should behave as if you had the flu: lots of bed rest, a little TV, few outings, and lots of tranquillity' (Colom & Vieta, 2006). Try not to schedule things for the evening, especially if they are stimulating, as they may keep you awake. Schedule calming activities such as sitting quietly in the garden, taking a relaxing bath, resting in dim light and doing relaxation exercises. Monitor yourself to see how your activities are affecting your mood. You can use the Mood and Activity Schedule to help you reduce your overactivity (see chapter 16). When your mood is more stable, restore your usual routine and regular sleep habits, but be sure to include calming activities and avoid overstimulation while you are recovering.

Prioritising goals and tasks

You may have many goals and tasks that you want to complete. Rather than increasing the activities in your usual schedule to achieve your goals, limit your activities. Here are some tips for cutting down:

- Be ruthless in eliminating or postponing goals that are not essential. It can be useful to enlist the help of someone you can trust to assist in prioritising them. List all the tasks or goals that are on your mind. Ask yourself: 'If I had to, could I do without a specific goal or what it is designed to achieve, or can that task or goal be postponed?' Extend your timeframes, so that some of the things you want to achieve now can be turned into longer-term goals, which will enable you to reduce your activity levels. If you can do without the task, cross it off your list; if you can postpone it, write 'P' next to it. Delegate tasks to give yourself permission to slow down. If you can delegate the task or a part of it, write 'D' next to it. Work out what are high, medium and low priority tasks or goals from what remains on your list. Prioritise goals around getting well before pursuing the rest.

- One way of eliminating goals is to assess each one to see whether it is realistic and whether you have considered the risks and dangers or negative consequences of carrying it out. The CARE tests in chapter 15 and the template on the website associated with this book can be helpful in checking out ideas or projects when you are going high.

- Structure forced breaks to give yourself some quiet time, and stick to regular times for meals, going to bed and waking up, despite your goals. Tom says: 'When I am doing a complicated assignment, I could carry on working all night, but I take regular breaks so that I don't become overstimulated and unable to sleep, and I try to stick to my usual routine.'

CHALLENGE UNHELPFUL THINKING EARLY

As we saw with depression, in cognitive behavioural therapy people are taught to identify, challenge and replace their unhelpful thinking with more helpful thoughts and actions. It is possible to use this cognitive restructuring with your hypomanic thinking, providing you are not too severely restless or agitated and are still able to consider other interpretations. There is little chance of arguing rationally with yourself once you are fully manic. Catching and challenging this kind of thinking early could help reduce the risk of negative consequences. To do this you need to be able to identify your unrealistic thinking. With practice at using cognitive restructuring techniques such as the Helpful Thought Summary, you can get to know your typical hypomanic patterns of thinking and helpful ways of responding. A more detailed guide to this cognitive restructuring may be found in *The Bipolar Workbook* by Monica Ramirez Basco (2006).

Being aware of your thinking patterns and typically helpful responses may assist you in distancing yourself and maintaining a more balanced perspective if you recognise unhelpful patterns arising. Cognitive restructuring is not meant to be used in isolation from other strategies for reducing your prodromes of hypomania or mania. This strategy helps to change your relationship to your hypomanic thinking so that you do not try anxiously to avoid it, pretend it is not there or simply follow its lead.

TYPICAL UNREALISTIC THINKING STYLES

People have identified a number of ways in which hypomanic thinking can become a bit illogical and unhelpful as you go up the bipolar roller-coaster. Feelings can be very powerful, and your judgments may be based on feeling elevated, excited or irritable rather than having much concern for the facts. Early changes to watch out for can be overly positive or overly negative thinking. For example, you may experience mostly positive thinking inter- rupted by irritable thoughts about others. Some people have much more negative thinking, especially when they are develop- ing dysphoric mania or mixed states. If this applies to you, we suggest you refer back to chapter 12, where there is more inform- ation about dealing with unhelpful depressed thinking.

Below are some of the typical unrealistic thinking styles that occur when thinking about yourself, others and the future.

Yourself

Your early thinking changes in hypomania may include progressively increasing self-confidence, and a focus on immediate gratification of your needs or the immediate achievement of your goals.

Overconfident thinking

You may develop beliefs about your personal ability, power and attractiveness that become increasingly unrealistic the more your mood rises—for example, 'I can drive very fast without having an accident' and 'I can pass this test without preparation'. This kind of thinking can lead you to try to achieve things that are unrealistic or result in difficult or even dangerous consequences, for example, risky investments and sexual indiscretions. You may speed up your activity level in order to achieve many of your valued goals and make your hypomania or mania worse. The object in challenging these overconfident thoughts is to try to find a more realistic version of your abilities that will not lead you astray.

'Extreme shoulds'

Thinking that involves extreme high standards about what you 'should' be like or able to do may lead to striving for unrealistic goals resulting in disappointment, disruption to routines and sleep, and increased illness. It can be helpful to recognise and replace such extreme expectations with those that take into account your strengths and weaknesses, realistic timeframes, resources, other demands and your health.

Overvaluing your needs and goals

As hypomania increases, people sometimes become focused on immediate satisfaction of their needs and goals. This may involve gratification of some desire like driving fast, buying that pair of shoes you cannot afford or phoning a friend in the middle of the night. It may also involve the need to achieve something without considering the effect on your health or on others. In a full episode of mania, your need for immediate gratification is more intense and harder to stop, and you can end up doing things that you bitterly regret. If you catch this thinking early enough, and consciously look for consequences and the effect of your choices on your health and on the people who matter, you may be able to prevent some of the damage. The strategies in the next chapter are designed to help you do this while your mood is not too severe.

Others and the world

You may see others or believe they see you in either a very positive or a very negative light. These extremes may signal that you are jumping to conclusions, and that it would be better to get all the facts before making any such assumptions. The following unrealistic thinking patterns with regard to others are common.

Mind-reading

Mind-reading involves jumping to the conclusion that you can read someone's mind so, for example, if a person smiles at you, you may assume that they are in love with you without knowing what they really think. Mind-reading can lead to disappointment, embarrassment and the disruption of relationships. To prevent such consequences arising, you may need to remind yourself that people behave the way they do for many reasons and that you may be mistaken about what they are thinking or their intentions. Think of the consequences of acting on a misinterpretation.

Personalising

Personalising involves jumping to the conclusion that something someone does or says, which is not directed at you, is really aimed at criticising or harming you—for example, 'You are trying to irritate me by stirring your tea in that way'. The awareness that you may be a little oversensitive, suspicious or defensive when you are hypomanic or becoming manic may help you to consider other explanations for people's behaviour. On the other hand, you may take personal credit for things that might have little or nothing to do with you—for example, 'My team won because I was playing'. This can lead to embarrassing consequences and contribute to manic grandiosity.

Blaming

You may find that you rush into judging and blaming others without considering contributing factors when you become hypomanic. This goes together with extreme thinking, so you set rigid standards that others 'should' be able to meet. An example of such an 'extreme should' is, 'You should always share my opinion or you are not my friend'. It also can be accompanied by harsh labelling in which the other person is stereotyped, such as 'You are an idiot'. Aiming for a more holistic view of the person and examining the unrealistic expectations and other factors that contribute to such situations can help to reduce this thinking.

Overestimating the goodness of the world

As hypomanic thinking increases, you may assume that others are trustworthy and supportive without really knowing what they are like. This can lead to unfortunate alliances. It can be helpful to dig a bit deeper rather than take things at face value.

The future

As optimism increases people see situations as less risky and underestimate dangers both for themselves and for others.

Optimistic fortune-telling

Hypomanic thinking can become very optimistic, so you might predict that the things you do will turn out wonderfully without really thinking them through. As this unrealistic optimism increases, the chances of taking on uncertain and even dangerous ventures rises. This is very different from realistic optimism, when you are hopeful about something without being blind to the difficulties involved. Knowing what the problems are may help you to make wise decisions and to address difficulties and adjust to situations that may not change. This can create a better future. The alternative to hypomanic or manic thinking does not necessarily mean doom and gloom. In challenging your thoughts and ideas as your mood is going up you may consciously look for the negative and the dangerous, for problems, but the aim of this self-examination is to provide a more balanced perspective and helpful actions for the future.

Under-estimating risks and consequences

The other side of this optimistic fortune-telling is a tendency to ignore the risks involved in doing something that is dangerous or can have negative consequences—for example, 'I bet my savings on a horse, but I am sure it will win the race'. For many people it is the under-estimation of risks and consequences when they are ill that results in some of the damaging consequences connected with manic behaviour. While you are not too manic and can still distance yourself from your thoughts, it can be helpful to realise that you may be under-estimating possible negative consequences and realistic difficulties and to consciously look for them.

KEY POINTS

- Catching warning symptoms early can be useful in preventing an episode of bipolar disorder or reducing relapse.
- Your doctor can help you to get the best from medication to prevent or reduce relapse and act on your behalf on the basis of prior arrangements, if things get worse.
- Other clinicians involved in your treatment can also boost your personal coping strategies.
- Reducing overstimulation and overactivity, and increasing your sleep can help prevent relapse, so you can return to your usual routines and sleep habits as soon as possible.

- Challenging rather than supporting hypomanic thinking helps to interrupt the activity cycle and reduce elevated or depressed thinking.
- Knowing that there are so many strategies for dealing with your symptoms of hypomania and mania may help you to feel less anxious when you recognise that you could be on the way up again.

15

PREVENTING DAMAGE AND BOOSTING YOUR COPING SKILLS

I am one step ahead of my mania by preventing its advance but also defending myself from its attack. **Ray**

Hypomania and mania can have unwanted costs. Apart from taking steps to prevent or reduce relapse, you can reduce damage connected to these mood states if they do occur. Many people find ways of minimising the potential damaging consequences resulting from these episodes of illness, consequences which can range from minor social indiscretions and inappropriate commitments, to serious disruptions to relationships and work, to financial repercussions and the tragic consequences of aggressive or suicidal behaviour.

Your own constructive coping skills may be reinforced by support from those close to you; in this chapter we suggest ways in which they can become your allies. Your strategies, combined with support from others, can act as a safety net to catch you as your mood escalates. You can assess whether you would like to include any of these ideas in your plan for preventing or reducing hypomania or mania (chapter 17).

DAMAGE CONTROL

Ideas for planning damage control when you are manic or hypo-manic include ways of managing money, avoiding risky sexual situations, remembering medication, avoiding alcohol and drugs, and dealing with risky or inappropriate ideas, irritability, anger and aggressive or self-destructive impulses.

Managing money

You may need to guard against spending sprees, gambling and wild investments. Here are some useful tips:

- Give your credit cards temporarily to someone you trust for safekeeping.
- Stay away from the shops.
- Don't surf the net if you are fond of online shopping.
- Avoid investing in the stock market.
- Put financial decisions on hold until you have fully recovered.

Avoiding risky sexual situations

People tend to get themselves into risky sexual situations when their mood is escalating, often with disastrous results for them-selves and their long-term relationships. If you know that you are prone to such risky encounters when going high, socialising only with people you know and can trust could be a helpful strategy. If you have a core person in your life who understands this, you can give them permission to give you a gentle reminder or offer you a lift home if they consider you are at risk of doing something you will later regret. Tell them to remind you that they are acting with your permission, according to your plan, so that you do not misinterpret their intentions.

Remembering medication

Sometimes when people become hypomanic or manic they see less of a need to take medication for their bipolar disorder, but skipping medication can leave you vulnerable to the full onslaught of untreated illness. It is wise to postpone any decision to stop or reduce medication until you have recovered.

Avoiding alcohol and drugs

Alcohol and recreational drugs may aggravate your escalating mood and inhibit self-control, making it more likely that you will act impulsively. To reduce this danger you may need to stay away from alcohol and drugs.

Risky or inappropriate ideas

A symptom of going high is that you have a flood of ideas, which can lead to loads of urgent new goals. In chapter 14 we discussed strategies for challenging the kind of unhelpful thinking that can encourage you to take risks and act on impulsive ideas. More ways of dealing with risky ideas, if you can catch them before your symptoms become too entrenched, include postponing major life decisions, drawing up an ideas list or carrying out the CARE test discussed below.

Postponing major life decisions

If you are going high, put on hold all important life decisions such as those about your relationships, work or finances. People with bipolar disorder make the best life decisions when they are well, and frequently end up regretting those they make when ill. Tell yourself that your certainty about decisions when you are going high might be due to your illness.

Ideas list

Using the website attached to this book, you can draw up a list of the ideas you have when going high and put it aside until you recover and are better able to evaluate their worth. This means that you will not waste the good ideas, and can put them into practice later in a way that will not overstimulate you.

CARE test

If you catch your ideas early when you're going high, you can subject them to the CARE test. CARE refers to Consequences,

Asking others, being Realistic and the Enough time test (there is a template for this on the website associated with this book). This involves recognising that due to your current mood state you probably need to examine your ideas and schemes more carefully.

Consequences

Look for the possible benefits and possible negative consequences that could result from your idea. Can it do harm to yourself or others? Can it result in regret or losses? (Scott, 2001). Something that has short-term benefits might have long-term risks, so you need to examine both the immediate and the long-term consequences. If you are unable to see negative effects, ask someone you trust for their opinion.

Asking others

Many successful people have personal advisers and consultants. Test any new ideas, schemes and plans on at least two other people in your support circle. If their opinion is different from yours, do not put your plan into action until your mood has had time to settle and you can reconsider the idea (Newman et al., 2002).

Realistic

Assessing whether your idea is realistic, possibly with the help of others, can help to avoid risky ventures.

- Firstly, is it realistic to put the idea into practice when you are symptomatic? Will it make your mood worse? What might be the consequences of making your mood worse? Consider postponing your idea until your mood is stable.
- Check if your thinking is unrealistic, risky or over-optimistic (chapter 14).
- In terms of resources, do you have the money, skills, people to help, training and experience to commit to doing this project?
- Look at the timeframe. Do you have enough time free of other goals so that putting your plan into action will not be disruptive?

Enough time

In reality, nearly all good ideas can be postponed. You can prevent damage and regret by waiting 48 hours, or preferably until you have had a few good nights' sleep, before making any decisions about acting on your ideas (Newman et al., 2002). If your idea has to be acted on immediately and there is a chance your mood is a little elevated, be suspicious that your judgment might not be as good as usual. It can be helpful to concentrate your energies on slowing down and reducing your warning signs while you are waiting. Include the idea on your ideas list so you can assess it when you have recovered.

Dealing with irritability and anger

We all feel irritable and angry at times. Anger is more extreme than irritability. Feelings can be intense and it can be hard not to express them impulsively. 'Even when the experience of anger is unpleasant, we often find it hard to give it up because we feel that if we do, the other person will somehow have won' (Jones et al., 2003: 79).

Irritability or anger can be a sign that you are feeling frustrated due to stress, or because someone has done something that doesn't fit with your expectations or needs or which simply offends you. If your irritability or anger is intense, persistent and not too discriminating in whom it targets, you should consider whether it might be a symptom of illness.

Irritability may accompany all the different mood states in bipolar disorder, including hypomania, mania, depression and mixed states. Irritability may hang around as a residual symptom between episodes of illness or be recognisable as a warning symptom.

Anger is often linked to mania as when people are manic, they develop a grandiose opinion of themselves, and can be very sensitive to anything they perceive as challenging their point of view or testing their patience. In this condition you may feel certain that your anger is justified, so it can be very difficult to use anger management strategies. Treating the illness reduces the anger. If you or those around you are scared that your anger is escalating, they need to leave the situation, and you need to get help immediately. Although not that common, violence can occur. Even when not so extreme, irritability and anger can disrupt relationships. There are several strategies you can use to reduce these symptoms before they become too severe.

Taking charge

If you consider that your irritability or anger is an ongoing symptom or a warning or early symptom of a bipolar episode, it may help to:

- seek treatment and put your relapse prevention plan into action if necessary.
- communicate to those who are close to you that this is part of your illness, so they do not misinterpret your irritability or anger as resulting from a flaw in your relationship, or think that you no longer care for them. This can also help them to take your behaviour less personally.
- give positive feedback when you can, as this can offset the times you respond with irritability and reassure those you care about. Positive feedback also encourages the other person to continue to do helpful things rather than the things that irritate you.
- work out some of the things that may trigger these feelings such as noise, arguments, socialising with certain people, discussions about money, changes in arrangements, work stress, clutter and traffic, and minimise the triggers.
- give permission when you are well for those close to you to contact your doctor, emergency department or even the police if your anger threatens to get out of control.

Ed has experienced irritability as an ongoing symptom of illness:

Irritability is an ongoing part of my life, and my partner and I have discussed it openly. I use medications to stabilise my moods, but when I do snap and criticise her for little things, she does not take it too seriously as she knows that it is a part of my illness. We are a close family and enjoy doing things together, and I show them that I really care. Sometimes I need to clarify when it is not the illness and I am really angry or concerned about something. Also, she makes an effort to do things to help me avoid some of the triggers of my irritability. Clutter and the kids' loud music set me off, and we both try to limit these in the house.

Defusing the situation

Other strategies that may help to reduce the intensity of these feelings and prevent damage in a particular situation, providing you are not too severely ill, are:

Time out

When you feel anger developing, or recognise that you are irritable, the best thing to do is to take time out and do something that relaxes you and helps you get a bit of distance from the situation. This time out provides space to calm down and decide how you want to act, instead of just expressing your irritability or anger and regretting it later. Examples are:

- leaving the room instead of responding, if necessary explaining that you will discuss things later or when you are well
- doing a relaxing activity to cool off, such as sitting outside or listening to soothing music
- counting to 10 before responding
- saying a few words to prompt yourself to stay calm such as 'Be calm, you will sort this out'
- saying 'stop' if you find it hard to stop thinking about what is making you angry and then trying to distract yourself by thinking or doing something pleasant.
- avoiding things such as alcohol as it can increase the possibility of acting impulsively on your angry feelings.

Gaining perspective

Considering the negative consequences of expressing your anger or irritability impulsively can be very useful. If you are well enough, you can check if your thinking about the other person is extreme or unrealistic before you express it. You can use the Helpful Thought Summary (chapter 12) to assist you with this. Unhelpful ways of thinking include blaming, exaggerating the bad, 'extreme shoulds', personalising things and mistaking feelings for facts.

When you feel irritable or angry with someone, it can be helpful to ask yourself if what they have done is really so terrible. What are the long-term consequences of what they have done? Does this person have good qualities too? What other factors contributed to the situation? Try and see things from their perspective as well. Are your expectations too high? Feeling that others should behave in the ways you would like them to become stronger when you become ill. Likewise, you may be more 'touchy', oversensitive to criticism and take offence more easily. Insight into this might help you to find a more realistic perspective.

Expressing your irritability or anger

Many people find that expressing their irritability or anger in writing, art or music helps to reduce its intensity. If you are not becoming elevated, so that exercise is not overstimulating, going for a run or having a good workout may decrease intense feelings.

Another way of expressing your anger or irritability, rather than bottling it up, is to share your feelings with someone you trust. Talking things through with someone who really listens can help put things into perpective. Be careful if you are becoming manic, because if someone starts giving you advice and telling you how your judgment is faulty, this could just increase your anger.

Once you have calmed down and can see things more clearly,

you might decide to express your concerns directly to the person concerned in a way that is assertive and respects your rights and those of the other person. This involves using ' I' statements and expressing clearly how the situation impacts on you and how it makes you feel without criticising the other person—for example, 'I am hurt that you did not consider my opinion when inviting them over for dinner, as I wanted to finish painting the spare room'. You can add positive requests for change—for example, 'I would feel less upset and angry if you consulted me before making an arrangement so we could work out arrangements that suit us both'. This is a way of channelling your anger to achieve constructive results.

If you consider that there is a problem between you that needs to be addressed, it is preferable to use the effective communication skills mentioned in chapter 19, such as active listening, making positive requests, finding workable compromises and problem-solving, to assist you in sorting it out. Postponing discussions of this nature until you are well can make things easier.

There are times when direct communication does not work. Expressing your anger by writing a letter that you do not send, or by confiding in someone you trust, can help to let off steam without doing any damage. Finding ways of enjoying life apart from this particular problem may make the situation easier to tolerate. Leaving a situation that regularly evokes anger in you and that is not likely to change might be an option, but such a major decision is best made when you are well.

Suicidal impulses

Suicidal impulses are generally considered to be a symptom of depression, but they can also occur as part of dysphoric mania. If you can see that you are developing suicidal impulses, get help immediately. You can put your Suicide Risk Prevention Plan into place (see chapter 13) and arrange with your close relative or friend to call your doctor or emergency department if you are in immediate danger.

Self-harm

Besides suicidal impulses, other forms of self-harm, including self-mutilation such as cutting, burning or scratching yourself, sometimes occur, particularly in depressive mixed states and dysphoric mania. These attempts at self-harm may be connected with your need to relieve emotional suffering. Medical treatment that reduces your other mood symptoms may be effective for self-harm as well. Psychologists may assist you in finding alternative strategies for reducing the intensity of your overwhelming feelings. If you consider that you are at risk of self-harm, contact your doctor.

IMPORTANT ALLIES

Just as with depression (chapter 11), close friends and relatives can be important allies in your efforts to prevent hypomanic or manic relapse and protect yourself from some of the consequences of your illness. They may play an important role, as sometimes it can be hard for people who are becoming ill, to recognise that they are ill, or to put strategies into place that are contrary to what their mood is telling them to do. Other people can make it easier to rest and slow down, too.

When becoming manic, it can be very difficult to give permission to others to help out; it is also difficult not to feel indignant or even hostile about their intervention in your affairs. For this reason it is wiser to discuss what suits you both, and to establish helping plans, when you are well. Not everyone has people whom they feel could be involved, while others may prefer to involve their clinicians rather than friends or family. Here are some ways others could be involved:

- Finding out about hypomania or mania and how you experience it in order to gain more understanding of your situation and not blame you for things you do when ill.

- Assisting you in recognising and monitoring symptoms.
- Assisting you in carrying out your constructive strategies to stay well and prevent relapse and possible damaging consequences. For example, helping you reach your doctor or making sure that the house is quiet, and taking over some of your tasks so you can rest.
- Giving you space but being nearby without being drawn into overstimulating discussions or arguments.
- Trying not to take your irritability personally if it is a symptom of illness.
- Not colluding with your developing episode by, for example, condoning or participating in risky behaviour, drug taking or drinking. Rather, they might consider stating their point of view calmly and quietly or postpone discussions on the subject until you are well.
- Not confronting or challenging you if you are irritable or aggressive; leaving to get help if they think you are at risk of becoming violent.
- Helping activate your suicide risk reduction plan early when necessary.
- Calling your doctor or the appropriate hospital emergency department or the police on your behalf if you get worse or are in danger of hurting yourself or others.
- Ask them, if absolutely necessary when you are too ill, to temporarily make urgent treatment decisions on your behalf and pre-empt what some of these decisions may be.
- After an episode they can give you time to recover and talk things through and problem solve around difficult consequences rather than criticise you.

KEY POINTS
- To some extent, hypomania, and particularly mania, can involve damaging consequences, and it can be helpful to prepare to minimise these consequences if you notice warning symptoms.

- These preparations include ways to manage your money, avoid risky sexual activities, remember medication, stay away from alcohol and drugs, deal with risky or inappropriate ideas, prevent irritability and anger from disrupting your relationships and protect yourself from suicide risk or self-harm.

- Friends and family can show that they care and value the person behind the illness and the efforts you are making to manage your illness. They can also assist you in practical ways to prevent and reduce relapse, and to minimise the damage that sometimes occurs. The extent of their involvement may differ depending on what suits you both and the severity of your symptoms.

16 MONITORING YOUR BIPOLAR DISORDER

To acquire knowledge, one must study; but to acquire wisdom, one must observe.

Marilyn vos Savant, *US* magazine columnist.

We all monitor and observe things without noticing. You may monitor the weather every day or how much leave you are accumulating at work. Monitoring is also a tool that can help you to keep a check on your illness so you can reduce symptoms and prevent relapse. It would be much easier if there were actual instruments to monitor symptoms of bipolar disorder as, for example, a thermometer measures fever. Nevertheless, you can develop your own ways of monitoring your illness and we present some suggestions in this chapter, such as the Daily Mood Chart and Mood and Activity Schedule. We suggest ways of monitoring your mood, triggers, warning signs, symptoms and treatment in order to gain more control over your illness. There are blank monitoring templates for you to fill in and print out for your personal use on the website associated with this book. We also discuss when monitoring is helpful and how to overcome some of its bothersome aspects.

DAILY MOOD CHART

Many people find it useful to have a broad overview of their moods and of particular symptoms such as anxiety, irritability, suicidal impulses, psychotic symptoms, sleep and weight changes, as well as their treatments and potential triggers, to assist them in managing their illness and making treatment decisions with their doctor. Table 16.1 is a comprehensive mood monitoring chart adapted from a mood chart developed through a Harvard research program (Sachs, 1993; Miklowitz, 2002) that enables you to record:

• Mood changes
• Specific symptoms
• Treatment: medications and counselling.
• There is also space to record daily stressors or triggers of illness. You can record beneficial and bothersome side effects of medications and your weight.

The chart contains space to record key information for an entire month on one page. It is a bit like travelling in an aeroplane and looking down to get a good picture of the land below. You will be able to see not only when your mood changes, but what factors contribute to the change. The chart gives a clear idea of how your treatment is helping, and what symptoms are persistent, making treatment decisions easier. Keeping track of vital symptoms such as sleep changes or suicidal impulses can empower you to take action before things get too bad. The numbers down the centre column in the mood rating area are the dates of the month, and you record your information corresponding to the relevant date.

Table 16.1, Madison's mood chart, is an example. Detailed instructions on how to fill in your own mood chart follow. You may notice that in this specific example, certain triggers such as a party and work deadlines disrupted Madison's sleep and contributed to her warning symptoms of mania. Using her observations on the chart, Madison eventually took action and managed to prevent relapse. She was also mindful that interpersonal stress affected her mood, and that she tended to become more irritable premenstrually.

RATING YOUR MOOD

The mood section of the monthly chart has sections labelled Depressed, Within Normal Limits (WNL) and Elevated. Under the Depressed and Elevated headings there are three levels of mood: mild, moderate and severe.

Start by rating your mood at day 1 according to the scale below.

- A score of –3 refers to severe depression, and a score of +3 to extreme happiness, elation or mania, or if you have bipolar II, to extreme hypomania.
- If mood is mixed, fill in two ratings, one in the Depressed section and the other in the Elevated section.
- If you experience more than one mood in a day, fill in the two ratings next to each other and make a note of your change in mood in the daily notes column.

To work out what mood you are in, it can be helpful to look at what your mood is usually like.

Within normal limits (WNL)

For some people with bipolar disorder, the distinction between their usual ups and downs when well is clearly different from the extreme moods they experience when ill, but for others the distinction is less clear. Your usual mood may be coloured by events, both positive and negative. For some, 'usual' may include some residual or mild symptoms that still interfere with your life and require attention, and would therefore be listed in the 'mild' section of the chart rather than within normal limits.

Some helpful distinguishing qualities of normal mood may be the following:

- Generally, during times of wellness, you think, feel and act in response to everyday events, the minor ups and downs. Such moods can occasionally be quite intense, for example, feeling sad when we have lost someone we love or feeling very happy when we have passed an exam, but these moods are not as enduring or extreme as mood changes in bipolar disorder. Thus, changes in mood are more short term and hinge on things occurring in our environment.
- When you are well, mood changes cause minimal disruption to everyday life, work and relationships compared to episodes of illness.
- When you are well, moods are usually not associated with long-term changes in sleeping, eating, libido or activity level.
- When you are well, it is easier to act in accordance with what is required in the situation, not just in accordance with what you feel inside.
- Others do not become as concerned over your mood.

In our experience, monitoring schedules work best when they are personalised so that you have a real sense of what is mild, moderate or severe for you. This is also something that you could work on with your clinician. As a guide, we provide some broad explanations of 'mild', 'moderate' and 'severe' below.

Mild

You may experience different types of mild symptoms, for example, very mild residual symptoms, or newly emerging

Table 16.1 Madison's mood chart

Month & year: May 2007
Monthly weight: 70 kg

(Circled dates indicate menstruation: days 6, 7, 8, 9, 10)

	Day 1	2	3	4	5	⑥	⑦	⑧	⑨	⑩	11	12
MOOD (place cross in box; Depressed – WNL – Elevated)												
Severe +3												
Moderate +2												
Mild +1					×	×	×					×
WNL (Mood not definitely elevated or depressed. No symptoms)	×	×	×	×				×	×	×	×	
Mild −1					×	×	×					
Moderate −2												
Severe −3												
SYMPTOMS (0 = none, 1 = mild, 2 = moderate, 3 = severe)												
Psychotic symptoms												
Suicidality												
Irritability	0	1	1	1	2	2	2	1	1	0	0	0
Anxiety	0	0	0	1	2	2	2	1	1	1	0	0
Hours slept last night	8	8	7	7	5	6	6	8	8	7	4	5
Daily notes					Argument with Trish			Sorted out problem with Trish			Terry's birthday, got to bed late	
Medication (enter name & number of tablets taken each day)												
Counselling	×							×				
—mg												
...mg												
....mg												
...—mg												
—mg												
Olanzapine 10mg												
Lithium.... 1000mg	4	4	4	4	4	4	4	4	4	4	4	4

Table 16.1 Madison's mood chart *Cont.*

Day		Notes					
13	x		5	0			4
14	x	Very busy day at work & forgot meds	5	0			−
15	x	Worked to meet deadline	3	0			−
16	x	Worked to meet deadline	3	0			−
17	x		4	0			4
18	x		5	0			4
19	x	Doing more, not sleeping call doctor	4	0			4
20		x	Thoughts racing	4	0		4
21		x	Saw doctor, prescribed meds to sleep	8	0		4 1
23	x	Relapse prevention plan for mania	10	0			4 1
24	x		11	0	x		4 2
25	x		12	0			4 1
26	x		8	0			4 1
27				8	0	x	4 1
28				9	0	x	4 1
29		Mood more stable and usual routine	7	0	x		4
30				7	0	x	4

Source: adapted from Sachs, 1993.

warning symptoms, or actual mild symptoms of an episode of illness. If your episode of bipolar disorder is mild, you will experience some symptoms, such as some sleep disturbance and slightly lowered or elevated mood, but they are not severe enough to cause much disruption to your life. You may notice subtle changes such as you cancel a few arrangements as you are becoming a bit socially withdrawn or, alternatively, make more arrangements than usual or spend more time at work if your mood is becoming elevated. Although you are still able to carry out your usual activities and commitments, if you recognise and monitor these changes (see page 208) and take action early you may be able to prevent relapse or reduce its severity. On the scale, mild is reflected as a -1 for depression or +1 for elevated mood.

Moderate

This refers to your mood state when it has progressed to an episode of illness but is not 'as bad as it can get' for you. Moderate is designated as −2 for depression or +2 for elevated mood. The symptoms you are experiencing are more intense and are noticeable to others. You may also experience difficulty in your usual day-to-day life, in your work or social relationships. You might be finding that you are experiencing conflict with others, or that your work performance is not what you are usually capable of.

Severe

This refers to the worst, most severe kind of mood state you experience, which seriously affects your daily life. This category is rated as a −3 for depression, or +3 for elevated mood.

OTHER SYMPTOMS

In addition to your general mood, if you are prone to suicidal thoughts, irritability, anxiety or psychotic symptoms, it helps to monitor them so that if necessary you can discuss them with your doctor and take action to reduce them. If you never have these symptoms leave the relevant box empty. Each of these is rated on a scale from 0 to 3, where 0 refers to absence of that symptom, and categories 1, 2 and 3 refer to mild, moderate and severe, as the symptoms relate to your experience. In general, mild symptoms are clearly more than usual, but don't cause much distress or impairment, moderate symptoms start to distress you or impair your functioning, and severe symptoms are very distressing and interfere greatly with your ability to function.

When considering suicidality, 0 refers to having no suicidal thoughts, 1 to having a few suicidal thoughts, 2 to thinking more about suicide and finding it harder to control suicidal thoughts and 3 to making plans about committing suicide, or wanting to act on suicidal thoughts. Mild suicidal symptoms need to be taken seriously (see chapter 13).

Sleep disruption is an important early warning sign of illness for many people, and it can also trigger an episode of illness. For this reason, it can be useful to estimate how many hours you slept last night when you are monitoring your mood.

TREATMENT

In addition to the symptoms discussed above, you can document your medication, blood tests and counselling sessions on your chart.

Medication

In the medication section, note the name of each medication and the number of tablets you have taken for each one. If you did not take medication on a particular day, draw a line through the box. You can note any beneficial or side effects of your medication in the daily notes section. Taking your medication regularly and observing how it is affecting your mood can help you to make informed treatment decisions and to get the best from your treatment.

Blood tests

For some medications (such as lithium and valproate), your blood levels will be monitored. Mark your chart with the initial of the medication (e.g. 'L' for lithium), the date the blood test was done, and your results.

Counselling

If you are seeing a counsellor or therapist, just place a cross on the dates of your sessions.

DAILY NOTES

The daily notes section enables you to record anything that you feel was significant in that day. This might include negative events and stressors; it could also include positive things that have happened. You can also use this section to describe symptoms in more detail or to mention side effects or good effects of your medications.

MENSTRUAL CYCLE

For some women there can be a relationship between moods and their menstrual cycle. You can monitor this simply by circling the dates of your period on the chart.

WEIGHT

There is space on the chart for you to record your weight each month. This can give you an idea if your weight is changing due to your mood or even as a possible side effect of certain medications. This should be done on the same date each month.

MOOD AND ACTIVITY SCHEDULE

If you would like to monitor your moods, anxiety, irritability, sleep and triggers more closely, you can use a Mood and Activity Schedule (see table 16.2) to:

- see what factors are triggering your moods or symptoms
- establish a balanced weekly structure or routine that helps keep your mood stable
- see how changes to your lifestyle affect your mood, such as going to the gym regularly, or starting work
- help you to carry out SMART goals that enrich your life without disrupting your mood (chapter 18).
- regulate your sleep, activities and stimulation if you notice warning or early symptoms of illness; for example, to help you to build up activities if you are becoming depressed or to slow down if you are becoming hypomanic or manic.
- assist you in getting back on your feet after an episode of illness.
- notice activities you enjoy so you can include them in your schedule while keeping well.

Common triggers of illness include stressful life events, the pursuit of positive achievements, disruption to activity level, routine and sleep, sensitivity to stimulation, drugs including alcohol, cigarettes and caffeine, relationship stresses, stopping medication, seasonal cycling and physical illness (chapter 9).

Rating your mood, anxiety and irritability uses the same scales as the daily mood chart above. Working out the hours you have slept can give you clues about sleep disruption, and it can be helpful to list specific sleep problems, such as not being able to fall asleep, waking early or restless sleep.

By filling in the major activities of the day and the approximate time you spent engaged in each, you will get a good idea of the type of activities you are doing, how much stimulation you are getting and how they are affecting your sleep and mood. The comments section enables you to record more detail and any relationships you have noticed between your activities, sleep, triggers, mood and symptoms. There are instructions and templates for filling in your own Mood and Activity Schedule on the website connected to this book.

John decided to fill out the Mood and Activity Schedule each evening to monitor his activities to see how they were affecting his mood, as illustrated in table 16.2.

In reviewing his Mood and Activity Schedule, John realised that although there were days when he did not feel like doing anything, if he gave into that feeling, he actually ended up feeling far worse by the end of the day. He discovered that work helped to structure his day, and that when he was not working he missed the structure, felt more lethargic and sometimes slept in the day, which made him feel a bit more depressed.

He realised that, even on his days off, having some planned activity was better for his mood. John realised that he enjoyed social contact, but did not participate in much social activity. His anxiety was also starting to interfere with his activities. John decided to build slightly more social activities and structure into his week, to try not to sleep or stay in bed during the day, and to monitor how this affected his mood. He also made up his mind to discuss his anxiety and depressive symptoms with his doctor and to activate his plan to reduce depressive relapse if his symptoms did not improve.

The schedule is like a diary or timetable that can give you insight and help you to control your moods and build a fulfilling life. Remember to notice things that have a good effect on your mood too. Sometimes you need to use the mood and activity Schedule for a while before the patterns and their influence on your mood become clear.

MONITORING YOUR PRODROMES

If you notice warning signs or symptoms, you can monitor them to see if they are subsiding or getting worse, and if you are

Table 16.2 John's mood and activity schedule

	Monday	Tuesday	Wednesday	Thursday	Friday	Saturday	Sunday
Mood : -3 to +3	0	0	0	0	-1	-1	-1
Irritability : 0-3	0	0	0	0	1	1	1
Anxiety : 0-3	1	1	1	1	2	2	2
Morning	Housework (2 hr) Gym (1 hr)	Work (6 hr)	Work (7 hr)	Gym (1 hr) Work (5 hr)	Supermarket (1 hr) Housework (2 hr) Cook meals to freeze for week (2 hr)	Computer games (3 hr) Slept in day (2 hr)	In bed until lunch time
Afternoon	Prepare for work meeting (1 hr)				Read (2 hr)	Watch sport (5 hr)	Read (4 hr)
Evening	Meet Paul for dinner (2 hr)	Watch TV (3 hrs) and read	TV (2 hr) Computer games (2 hrs)	Internet (2 hrs) Watch TV (2 hr)	TV (2 hr)	TV (4 hrs)	TV (5 hr)
Stressor/triggers	Uncomfortable alone at gym				Anxious at supermarket	Not much structure today. Slept during day	Felt more down
Hours slept	8	8	8	8	10	11	5
Comments	Enjoyed dinner with Paul. Maybe plan more social activities					Sleeping in day and lack of structure makes me more tired and bored	Planned to go to gym but anxious to go alone. Anxiety gets in the way of doing things. The less I do the more lethargic I feel

developing more symptoms. Some people find this helpful, as what they might do in response to mild early warning signs may differ from their strategies when their warning signs become worse or when they develop early symptoms of an episode. For example, if you have been taking your usual medication and your mood has been stable but then things get a bit frantic at work and you find yourself feeling slightly more energetic and restless than usual, you might take action early and decide to slow the pace and restore your routine, have quiet times and keep an eye on your mood. You may see an improvement as you eliminate the things that are triggering your mood. However, if these early mild changes persist or increase, and more warning symptoms of mania appear, such as finding it difficult to sleep, you may need to implement additional strategies to reduce your chances of full relapse.

There are templates of the 'monitoring warning signs' table for depression, mania and mixed states on the website associated with this book. As an example, here is Fred's 'warning signs of depression' table (see table 16.3 below). The idea of the table is to fill in the warning sign you are experiencing in the first column. Fill in the date and place an X on the days when it occurs. Use one X for when the symptom is mild, two Xs if it gets worse. If you have other warning signs you can add them in the same way. Having a list of your typical warning signs of an episode is helpful as you can simply fill in X's if they occur.

Table 16.3 Fred's warning signs of depression

Date	7/8	8/8	9/8	10/8	11/8	12/8	13/8
List warning symptoms:							
No energy	x	x	x	xx	xx	xx	xx
Cancelling plans			x	x	xx	xx	xx
Irritability					xx	xx	xx
Crying							

When to monitor

For some people monitoring their mood becomes like having a shower: they do it daily without even thinking. It is a habit. Knowing when to monitor is about finding a balance whereby you can keep an eye on your illness so that you notice changes early but do not focus on it all the time to the extent that you are less able to participate in and enjoy life. Some people monitor their moods or specific symptoms to find out if a new treatment is working. If you are making any changes to your lifestyle, if you are under stress or if there are triggers that might set off your symptoms, it is a good idea to increase your monitoring and to be more vigilant about watching for warning or early symptoms. Changes in mood may signal that you are becoming ill and necessitate an increase in monitoring until your mood settles again. Some people find it helpful to continue to monitor their mood at least every other day for a few weeks after an episode is over until they have re-established their healthy lifestyle.

Overcoming common barriers

There are a number of common barriers to monitoring your bipolar illness. Below is a list of barriers and tips for overcoming them.

'I know it's a good idea, but I can't be bothered'

If the task of monitoring seems too daunting, start small. Decide what is most important to monitor at that particular time, so that you are not burdened with trying to monitor everything at once. For example, you may decide to spend a few months monitoring the effects of a new medication, or decide to monitor your sleep if it is becoming disrupted, and to look out for other symptoms and triggers that may be linked to sleep disruption. You might find it convenient to use the templates on this book's website to record information. They can help you set aside a regular time for monitoring, so you are less likely to forget to do it.

Reminder of illness

For some, monitoring seems too much of a reminder of their bipolar disorder. If monitoring makes you feel uncomfortable or anxious, remind yourself that it is a way of gaining more control over your illness so that you can get the most out of life.

'Hard to pick what mood I'm in'

For some people, getting in touch with moods can be difficult. As Jacquie expressed it, 'It can be hard to know what is normal and what is up when I am happy: am I happy and that is normal—or is it because I am going high?'

Chapter 10 highlighted some tips on identifying when you are becoming symptomatic. Asking a trusted friend or exploring this more with your doctor can help make identifying your mood a little easier.

KEY POINTS

- A daily mood chart can give you a good overview of how things are going, and allow you to monitor specific areas of concerns such as medications, suicidality and other symptoms and stressors.
- The Mood and Activity Schedule provides a useful way of monitoring the effect of your activities and sleep on your mood. It can also be used to plan activities or a routine that helps to reduce relapse if you have warning signs, or to reduce ongoing mild symptoms and can help maintain a healthy lifestyle.
- The 'monitoring warning signs' table helps to keep an eye on your warning signs so you know when you need to use additional illness management strategies.
- There are useful tips about when to use monitoring and overcoming common barriers to monitoring.

17 PLANNING TO PREVENT OR REDUCE RELAPSE

> My plan is a safety net that I have in place. There are many
> points at which I can take charge of my illness when I need
> to, so, besides taking my medication and maintaining my
> lifestyle, I worry less about my bipolar disorder and get on
> with my life. **Janet**

Many people keep well by using prescribed medications and
strategies to maintain a healthy lifestyle. In addition, having
personal plans tailored to preventing relapse of the particular types
of episodes you experience may help you to gain more control
over your bipolar disorder. These plans can include strategies you
consider helpful in dealing with your triggers and warning and
early symptoms. There are also things you can do to reduce
symptoms if things do get worse, and to decrease the negative
consequences resulting from an episode of illness. Many people
find that having relapse prevention or reduction plans makes the
prospect of relapse a little less worrying.

In this chapter we look at developing plans for reducing the
risk of relapse that people can adapt to suit their specific

circumstances. We also discuss overcoming some of the obstacles to implementing these plans when you need them most.

WHY DEVELOP PLANS?

These plans focus on using information about your illness, and what helps to increase your control over it. The advantage of having an action plan to prevent or reduce relapse is that it is a summary of key strategies that you have organised in advance to some extent. It is particularly helpful to decide on strategies when you are well and thinking clearly. This means that when you are stressed and facing high-risk situations, or becoming symptomatic, you do not need to start from the beginning or work things out and make lots of decisions. Having a plan can also be a time-saver when you need to act promptly before symptoms become too entrenched.

TIPS FOR DEVELOPING PLANS

Here are a few tips about developing action plans:

- Develop separate written plans for the different types of mood episodes that you experience.
- Include what you know about your typical triggers and warning or early symptoms, and the constructive strategies you have discovered for dealing with them.
- A few core strategies may be more effective than lots of complicated instructions.
- Be specific when including a constructive strategy, such as 'Tim to help me monitor symptoms when my mood is going down', rather than 'Ask others to help me monitor symptoms'.
- Strategies need to be practical and realistic. For example, suddenly expecting yourself to run five kilometres a day to

reduce warning symptoms of depression can be unrealistic if you are not fit enough to do it.

- In your plan, aim to respond to your symptoms as early as possible, as it can be easier to respond constructively when symptoms are not too entrenched. Also include what to do in case symptoms do get worse.

- Sometimes different people can provide different kinds of support. For example, a neighbour might help with your children but your mother could collect them after school. Your clinician may give you a prescription for certain medication if you are becoming manic or arrange for admission to a particular hospital if necessary. It is important to negotiate this involvement with the individuals concerned.

- Make sure you have up-to-date contact details for everyone involved in your plan and for the hospital emergency department. It is useful to have alternative contacts in case someone is unavailable.

- Give the key people involved a copy of the plan. Some people have found it useful to ask others who are central to the plan to sign it, which makes it like a contract they can rely on.

- Leave your plan within easy reach if you should need it.

- Regard your plan as a work in progress, and amend it as you learn more about your illness and ways of coping with it.

I have developed a list of my warning signs of mania and an action plan, which I keep in the drawer next to my bed. I gave copies to my best friend, Jane, and my doctor, and those two people have permission to tell me if they notice warning signs. Also in the plan, I have arranged to give Jane my credit cards for safekeeping until I feel better, and for her to call my doctor if I become too ill. Jane offered to run a few errands for me if my doctor gives me extra medication to slow me down. **Elizabeth**

DEVELOPING YOUR PLANS

You may already have a number of constructive strategies you use to prevent or reduce your episodes of illness. There are more suggestions in the other chapters of this book, and you can find templates that you can use to develop your own relapse prevention plans on the website associated with this book.

If you have a tendency to become suicidal, having a separate Suicide Risk Prevention Plan to rely on can be very helpful (see chapter 13).

Each person needs to develop plans that suit their situation. Dan's plans for preventing or reducing his depressive and manic relapses provide examples of developing personal plans. Dan is married to Sandra. They have a five-year-old daughter, Terry. Dan runs a small but successful consultancy business from home, and Sandra is a journalist. He was diagnosed with bipolar I disorder ten years ago and has since developed and refined his plans for preventing or reducing relapse (see figures 17.1 and 17.2). Although 'breakthrough' depressive episodes occur from time to time, Dan has not had a manic episode for the past five years. He leads a reasonably healthy lifestyle and considers that finding the right mood stabiliser has made an enormous difference to both his life and his relationship with his wife.

Figure 17.1 Dan's plan for preventing or reducing depressive relapse

---

1. Useful information

Health care details

Medicare number: 4783254681

Pension card number: 902654682

Health insurance: 82963 BBB Health Insurance

continued

Clinicians' contact details
(*List more than one name if possible in case your doctor is unavailable or if you wish to contact your caseworker or psychologist.*)

Doctor's name: Dr Joyce	Phone number: 2378 9398
	Doctor's emergency number: 0487 297 864
Other clinician's name: Dr Pomelo	Phone number: 2893 0407
	Doctor's emergency number: 0421 534 741
Hospital emergency department	Phone number: 999

Key support people

Name: Sandra Jones (wife)	Phone numbers: 2963 8465 or 0483 756 054
Name: Myra Til (mother)	Phone numbers: 2893 7546
Name: George Til (father)	Phone numbers: 0473 954 065
Name: Tim Burt	Phone numbers: 0489 728 653

2. Managing triggers

Triggers to monitor
(*List the high-risk situations or triggers that might lead to depressive symptoms.*)

1. Work stress and too many deadlines
2. Arguments with Sandra
3. Cycle into depression from mania

Ways to manage triggers
(*List the things that you can do to manage these triggers and how others can support your strategies.*)

continued

1. Monitor my mood and warning symptoms if triggers present.
2. Do pleasurable and relaxing things.
3. Prioritise work goals, and delegate overload.
4. Remind myself about unrealistic 'extreme shoulds' that tell me I should always get everything done perfectly.
5. Check that work goals do not interfere with sleep, and take regular breaks.
6. Use good communication skills and problem solving to sort out arguments and do enjoyable things with Sandra.
7. After manic episode, restore routine, reorganise duties to avoid overload and do not neglect pleasurable experiences.
8. Remember mania is not my fault and challenge negative thinking about myself.

Things not to do
(*List the ways you may sometimes manage triggers that are not helpful or make things worse.*)
1. Don't use alcohol to relieve stress, although it makes everything feel better initially, as I feel more depressed next day.
2. Don't give up walking the dog every day when stressed, as exercise clears my mind.

3. Managing warning or early symptoms
Warning/early symptoms to monitor
(*List your typical warning or early symptoms so you can intervene early.*)
1. Don't enjoy things I used to anymore.
2. Tired and lethargic.
3. Worry about little things.

Ways to manage warning or early symptoms
(*List the things that you can do to prevent or reduce relapse if you*

continued

*notice warning or early symptoms and ways key people can
support your strategies.)*

1. Monitor mood and symptoms and make appointment for assessment with Dr Joyce.
2. Maintain usual activities, but if they become too overwhelming, prioritise and divide into smaller achievable goals.
3. Maintain regular sleep patterns.
4. Do something from my pleasurable activity list each day.
5. Use Helpful Thought Summary and make an appointment with my psychologist, Dr Pomelo, to help manage the worry.
6. Discuss warning symptoms with Sandra, and go for drives and walks together.
7. If I start to feel suicidal, put suicide risk prevention plan into operation.

Things not to do
*(List the things that you may sometimes do to cope with warning
or early symptoms that may make your symptoms worse.)*
Watch out for a tendency to:

1. ignore my warning symptoms
2. sleep all day
3. make life changing decisions
4. keep my suicidal impulses a secret

4. Being prepared if things get worse
(List what you or others can do if your symptoms get worse.)

1. Activate Suicide Risk Prevention Plan.
2. Call the doctor and schedule an earlier appointment and frequent monitoring appointments.
3. Call Tim to help extend work deadlines and do overload.
4. Ask parents to fetch Terry from school and whether she can stay with them until Sandra gets home from work.

continued

5. Make sure I do something every day, and gradually try to restore usual activity level. Use my Reasons for Wanting to Reduce Relapse list to help with this (see below).

6. If my mood becomes more severe or I am very suicidal, ask Sandra to contact Dr Joyce or his usual locum and take me to Rose Clinic for admission.

7. If I am admitted to hospital, my parents can help Sandra look after Terry and do the shopping.

Figure 17.2 Dan's plan for preventing or reducing manic relapse

(*Dan listed his health care details and the contact details of his clinicians and key support people.*)

1. Managing triggers

Triggers to monitor

(*List high-risk situations and triggers that might lead to manic symptoms.*)

1. Lots of socialising and celebrations.
2. Working for many hours with no breaks to meet deadlines.
3. Jet lag when flying to a later time zone.

Ways to manage triggers

(*List the things you can do to manage these triggers and how others can support your strategies.*)

1. Monitor mood and warning symptoms daily if triggers present.
2. Reduce the number of social arrangements and the duration spent celebrating so that it's easier to maintain regular sleep habits.
3. Keep to my usual routine.
4. Take breaks and do relaxing things even if I have deadlines.
5. Gradually go to bed earlier and earlier the week before I travel.

continued

Restore usual sleep habits in the time of my current location as soon as possible. Plan restful activities in my schedule to reduce over-stimulation in the new country.

Things not to do
(*List the ways you may sometimes manage triggers that are not helpful or make things worse.*)
1. Watch out for tendency to do more, make more arrangements after parties and excessive working to meet deadlines.
2. Don't sacrifice sleep patterns and routine in pursuit of goals.

2. Managing warning or early symptoms of hypomania or mania
Warning/early symptoms to monitor
(*List your typical warning or early symptoms so that you can intervene early. Some people find they have early and later warning symptoms when becoming manic.*)
1. Early warning symptoms: more energy and take on more projects than when I am well.
2. Late warning symptoms: same as early signs but also can't sleep and not tired and start going to pub to gamble.

Ways of managing warning or early symptoms
(*List the things that you can do to prevent or reduce relapse if you notice warning or early symptoms and ways key people can support your strategies.*)

Responding to early warnings
1. Monitor mood and prodromes daily and ask Sandra to assist with monitoring.
2. Call doctor and make appointment.
3. Take regular breaks while working, stick to a daily structure and make no commitments to new projects until I feel better.
4. Reduce social arrangements.
5. Include relaxing activities, like staying home and listening to music.
6. Exclude stimulating activity before bed. If find it hard to sleep

continued

do relaxation exercise and if necessary take prescribed medication to help me sleep.

Responding to late warnings

1. Take prescribed medication to slow down and sleep, and stick to regular sleep times.
2. Give credit cards, laptop and car keys temporarily to Sandra.
3. Use calming music, walks or long baths to help slow down.
4. Hand over some work to Tim and extend other work deadlines.
5. If I am a bit sedated from extra medication, arrange for parents to fetch Terry from school and look after her until Sandra gets home.

Things not to do
(*List the things that you may sometimes do to cope with warning or early symptoms that may make your symptoms worse.*)

1. Deny symptoms and go with the activity flow.
2. Find reasons not to take prescribed medications.
3. Make decisions about work or that involve money.
4. Go to the pub to gamble.

3. Being prepared if things get worse
(*List what you or others can do if your symptoms get worse.*)

1. Sandra or I will arrange urgent appointment with Dr Joyce or his locum.
2. If at home, take medication and try to rest, and see doctor more often.
3. If hospitalisation is required, I wish to be admitted to Rose Clinic.
4. Parents have offered to help Sandra with Terry.

IMPLEMENTING YOUR PLAN

Implementing your plan is often just a matter of following the strategies, but sometimes you may need to troubleshoot difficulties. Even the best plans may have teething problems, and some of them can be avoided by problem solving if unforeseen difficulties occur, such as finding that your doctor is on leave. People who have lived with bipolar disorder for a long time recommend using plans as a guide and being flexible rather than expecting that things will always work perfectly. Your developing symptoms themselves can make implementing your plans a bit harder. Here are some recommendations for dealing with mood-related difficulties when implementing your plans.

'It's too difficult to get going'

People sometimes find that early depressive symptoms such as lethargy, poor concentration, worry and negative thinking undermine their efforts to implement their plan. Prioritising your action plan as something that you need to put into place, and enlisting the help of a key person, can make things easier. Assigning a special time to do the things in your plan, breaking them into smaller steps, completing one step at a time and rewarding yourself afterwards may help.

'My feelings tell me to do the opposite to my plan'

Putting plans into practice may mean going against your current feelings. As Ryan explained when he was becoming depressed: 'I did not feel like visiting Carol or anyone else, but there were a few other people there. I did not have to do much, and they were really funny. It was relaxing, and I felt a little less flat afterwards.' This is also true when you become hypomanic, when your feelings tell you to speed up and keep going but you need to slow down to reduce your growing mania.

If you can recognise what is going on and take action early enough, it is easier to act contrary to these feelings. Acknowledging these feelings and recognising that they are part of your bipolar disorder and not who you are may help you to act contrary to the dictates of your illness. Remind yourself that you are more than your feelings. Looking 'at' your feelings rather than 'through' them may assist you in finding a bit of relief and gaining the necessary distance to act to reduce your depression or hypomania (Marra, 2004). Some people explain that they experience this as linking up with that part of themselves that stands back, monitors things, and looks after their long-term interests when they are becoming ill.

It can be harder to maintain this distance when you are becoming hypomanic or manic, as you may easily lose insight into the fact that you are becoming ill, which is why it is so important to take action early. For this reason, people recommend having a key person who can be an ally and help you monitor your warning signs and use your helpful strategies. It is important that they provide this support early, as you may stop listening to their advice and get irritable as your mania progresses.

Some people find that weighing up the costs of being ill against the benefits of being well helps them to put their plan into practice. It can be helpful to use this assessment to develop a Reasons for Wanting to Reduce Relapse list (see the website associated with this book). You can develop this list when you are well, and keep it handy to remind you about why you want to go against what your illness is telling you to do, and take action to get well when you are developing an episode of illness. Your reasons may differ depending on the type of episode.

Weighing up the long-term costs and consequences of being ill against the benefits of being well can motivate you to implement your action plan to prevent hypomania or mania. Such delays may result from uncertainty about whether you would prefer to go with the seductive hypomania or mania or to control it. Mania has many potential consequences, including those linked to relationships and financial security and your basic safety. Hypomania for people with bipolar II is inevitably linked to depression. Delays in taking action to prevent relapse can be costly.

Worry and denial

Worry about relapse when you notice warning symptoms can lead to denial on the one hand or anxiety on the other.

Denial can mean that you ignore warning symptoms when you have the best chance of preventing or reducing relapse. Coming to terms with your illness and knowing that there are many helpful strategies for managing it may ease these concerns.

It is normal to be concerned about relapsing, but this concern can become excessive and transform into an avalanche of rumination about your mood, your illness and the future. This may get in the way of carrying out your action plan. Specifying exactly what is worrying you may give you clues about ways of reducing excessive anxiety. For example, if you are worried about getting behind at work, you may be able to prioritise tasks, delegate them, postpone them or extend deadlines. It can be helpful to deal with this worry with the assistance of your clinician, who can provide a more objective perspective and help you to sort out realistic concerns. This will include ways of managing if things do get worse in your relapse prevention plans and may alleviate some of this anxiety.

KEY POINTS

- The prospect of relapse can be daunting. It is helpful to prepare specific and practical strategies ahead of time when you are well. This way you can activate your plans when you notice triggers, warning or early symptoms, to prevent relapse from happening or to reduce its severity and its consequences.

- There are a number of things to consider when developing these plans, such as the successful strategies you already use, and what has been unhelpful or made things worse.
- You are not alone in trying to prevent or reduce relapse and its effect on your life. Your doctor and trusted others can participate in your plans.
- Sometimes you may need to troubleshoot problems that interfere with your plans and deal with mood-related issues that get in the way of implementing these plans. Usually the earlier you apply your strategies, the easier it can be to control your illness.
- It is important to see your plan as a work in progress. As you learn more about your illness and what works and, as people in your support system change, you may need to update your plan.
- You can use the templates on www.eburypublishing.co.uk/bipolar and the suggestions in this book to develop plans to prevent and reduce relapse of your bipolar episodes.

18 MAINTAINING A HEALTHY LIFESTYLE

To stay well, most people with manic depression make some lifestyle changes. These may be quite small changes such as remembering to take medication and being mindful about sleep. However, some make significant changes such as adopting a quieter lifestyle in a rural community and changing jobs.

Sarah Russell, *A Lifelong Journey*, 2005:83.

Your lifestyle may affect your stress levels, and help keep triggers and symptoms of bipolar disorder to a minimum. This can leave you free to focus on other aspects of your life. You can make choices about your lifestyle that can help you to adapt to your bipolar disorder and live a fulfilling life. It is important not to make any major lifestyle decisions like resigning from work or ending a relationship when you are ill, as you may not see things the same way when you are well. Rather, take time out to get well, and decide on things when you have been well for a while. In this chapter we look at ways of keeping well and enriching life. We also discuss other good habits such as exercise, stress management, a healthy diet and avoiding toxic substances.

KEEPING AN EYE ON YOUR BIPOLAR DISORDER

Keeping well involves finding a balance between keeping an eye on your illness and focusing on your life, in a way that does not detract from your health but allows you to enjoy life. Some people experience a few ongoing symptoms between episodes of bipolar disorder. Often depressive symptoms are most persistent and disruptive; the treatment, support, activity and thinking strategies mentioned in the chapters on reducing depressive relapse may be helpful in reducing your residual symptoms as well.

It is not necessary to be constantly preoccupied with your bipolar disorder when you are well. Nevertheless, taking medications regularly and scheduling regular check-up appointments with your doctor and keeping an eye on your mood, triggers and warning symptoms will give you a chance to attend to your illness while getting on with life. You can always implement your relapse prevention plans if necessary.

'Sleep and mood are virtually joined at the hip' (McManamy, 2006:167). As sleep disruption can so easily trigger mood episodes, part of your healthy lifestyle might include having a general daily activity structure that is not overstimulating, and that helps you to maintain regular activity levels during the day so you can ensure regular sleep habits. Some obvious things that can disrupt your sleep include shift work, jet lag and work stress, and difficult choices about these matters sometimes need to be made. If your sleep or routine has been disrupted, and you are feeling a bit hyped up or excited, rather than taking that as a signal to race around and get lots done, make sure you take things easy and restore your usual sleep and activity patterns. There are tips for maintaining healthy sleep habits and stimulation levels, and an activity schedule, in chapter 9.

ENRICHING DAILY LIFE

There are many ways to enrich daily life, including enjoying relationships and doing enjoyable and meaningful things.

Relationships

Relationships don't always bring enjoyment, but when they are good, they are rewarding and promote your health. There are ways of dealing with interpersonal problems and maintaining good relationships (see chapter 19).

Family, friends, work colleagues and people you meet through your various interests all provide the opportunity for social interaction. Some people enjoy participating in Internet chat-rooms for people with bipolar disorder, or attending meetings and functions with their local peer support group. People have commented that they have felt accepted and valued by these groups, and that, apart from receiving help when it has been needed, giving help to others and having the opportunity to share their knowledge and experience is meaningful.

They also offer words of caution, in that not all strategies for managing bipolar disorder suit everyone, so what works for one person in the group might not work for the next person. People's advice when they are ill may not be as sound as their advice when they are well. Personal experience is valuable, but there are times when people need medical advice no matter what their illness. With these cautions in mind, it is clear that other people with bipolar disorder and their families are a valuable resource. These networks can also create good friendships. They also provide valuable services including employment, housing, drop-in services, advocacy, activity programs and family-to-family support. To find local support groups, you can contact your national or local mental health organisations; we also have listed some Internet support organisations on the website associated with this book.

Participating in life

Participating in life can involve activities of different kinds, including those that involve duty, stress relief or pleasure, and those that give you a deep sense of satisfaction because they express your talents or are in harmony with your values and what is important to you in life. A one-sided emphasis on achievement can lead to setting unrealistic goals and drive you to chase your goals in a way that is disruptive to your health. At the other extreme, sitting back and doing very little can make you feel unfulfilled and lethargic. Thus it can be helpful to pursue realistic meaningful goals in a way that enhances satisfaction but does not interfere with your health.

As too much goal-pursuit can contribute to the spin into mania and hypomania, people sometimes find it helpful to consciously take regular breaks, relax and stick to their sleep patterns when planning timeframes for achieving a goal. To stay on track when you get home after stimulating activities, give yourself time to relax and unwind. The Mood and Activity Schedule (chapter 16) can also help you work out whether what you are doing to achieve your goals is disrupting your mood.

Thinking of your goals as journeys can be a useful metaphor. This emphasises that it is not just getting there and achieving the final goal that is central, but that the process of achieving the small steps along the way and making the most of the journey enriches your life.

Your self-esteem can be eroded by disruptive episodes of illness and setting unrealistic goals. Achieving manageable goals and acknowledging these achievements can enhance self-esteem and fulfilment.

Setting SMART goals

The acronym SMART can help you set goals that are realistic and not too stressful in your current situation. You can check to see whether your goal is Specific, Measurable, Achievable, Realistic and Timely. There is a template on the website connected to this book for you to use to check your goals are SMART and to assist you in carrying them out in a way that is not disruptive to your health.

Specific

Your goal needs to be specific so that you know when you have achieved it. For example, the goal 'I want to get fitter' is not specific enough. 'I plan to go swimming three times a week' is clearer.

Measurable

Having a goal that is measurable enables you to plan what you want to do and to know when you have achieved your goal. For example, 'I plan to go swimming three times a week' could be put in even more measurable terms, such as 'I plan to swim twenty laps of the local pool three times a week'.

Achievable

When setting your goal, it is important that it is a goal that can be reached. You may need to examine the barriers to achieving your goal. Your plan to swim twenty laps three times a week might not be possible if you have not exercised for some time. Setting a lower target of five laps may be more within reach when starting.

Big or long-term goals may need to be divided into smaller, more achievable steps. The long-term goal of completing a university degree can be easily broken down to smaller achievable goals, like completing one or two subjects in a semester. This way the longer-term goal does not seem so daunting. In addition, you will get a sense of satisfaction from achieving the steps along the way.

You may want to distinguish between short-term goals that can be achieved within a day to a week or two, medium-term goals with timeframes of a few weeks or months, and long-term goals that take months or years to achieve. Managing to achieve short-term goals can show you that you are capable of doing what you set out to do. Having longer-term goals that are meaningful to you can provide a sense of purpose and direction in life.

You may also need to consider that what you hope to achieve involves a certain amount of risk and examine what is at stake. For example, if your goal is to pursue a get rich quick scheme you may need to weigh up the chance of landing up in debt rather than with the fortune you hope for.

Realistic

In setting a goal that is realistic, you are asking yourself how practical you are being. This can be hard when you want the answer to be 'yes'. Everyone has limitations on what goals are viable. To set a realistic goal you need to consider what resources, skill and experience are needed to achieve the goal. Then, weigh up not only your ability and skills and the resources you have, but also consider possible constraints such as symptoms of illness, current circumstances, what time you have available and so on. For example, you might consider your current situation and decide that it is unwise to leave a good job for a more glamorous position that is exciting but very pressurised and time intensive, and assumes that you have experience that you actually don't have. Dividing your goal into steps and seeing if each step is realistic can give you a good idea of whether to pursue this goal or not.

It may be that although a particular goal is something important, other goals need to come first. You may need to set the goal of getting bipolar symptoms more under control first, or obtaining certain resources or skills, before the ultimate goal is achievable. Trying to pursue too many goals at once is unrealistic, and can be bad for your health, so it is essential to prioritise which goals to pursue in the time available.

If you still have some symptoms of bipolar disorder that get in the way when you are well, or are prone to rapid cycling, it may be necessary to adjust your expectations to take this into account. Setting smaller and more manageable goals may be helpful. This is important to consider when you have recently emerged from an episode of illness. Some people find it helpful just to make a start and set a small achievable goal rather than to rush and take care of all the accumulated demands. It is the 'small triumphs' that can be healing at these times and while you are ill (Deegan 1994:154).

Timely

Setting yourself a timeframe can help keep you motivated, because it means that there is an end point. Timeframes need to have flexibility and to take into consideration the other things happening in your life, including any other goals you have already set. If you find deadlines stressful, your timeframes need to be less rigid, and you may need to allow for extra time so that you do not feel too pressured. You will need to adjust these timeframes if you become ill.

Carrying out your goal

Once you have divided your goal into steps you can plan how to proceed with the first step, implement your plan and evaluate how it is going. If you experience difficulty, getting assistance, problem solving, changing the timeframe or dividing a goal into even smaller steps may help. There are times when you might need to give up a goal that is important to you, and this can be difficult. A good idea when you are trying to find alternative goals is to consider your strengths and values, and to find realistic goals in harmony with them. In this way, even if you are not doing what you were doing before, you will be heading in a direction that is important to you.

Find something that you enjoy

Finding something that you enjoy doing, that gives meaning or purpose to your life, can help you live well with bipolar disorder.

Participating in life in a way that expresses some of your strengths and what you value without making you ill can be very fulfilling. John McManamy explains that writing helped him to reclaim his life with bipolar disorder:

> Writing is what helped bring me back from the dead. For me, it is a healing activity. If I were a basketball player, I'd be shooting hoops; if I were a gardener, I would be out with the petunias. Healing is about finding something that makes you feel alive (McManamy, 2006:344).

Doing things you value in everyday life, for example, going for a regular walk with a friend, playing with your pets and participating in a cause you believe in, or doing work or a hobby that you love, are some of the many things that can enrich life. We are all different, and it is about finding those things that enrich your life.

Other good habits

You can develop other good habits such as doing regular exercise, managing stress, eating a healthy diet and avoiding toxic substances.

Exercise

Natural body chemicals (endorphins) released during exercise have stress-reducing properties. Exercise has also been found to reduce depression and anxiety, although it might make you overstimulated if you already have symptoms of mania or hypomania. It also has other health benefits such as protecting you from heart disease and diabetes. It is sensible to build up an exercise routine gradually and to have a medical check-up before embarking on a new course of exercise. Exercising with a friend can help you to get going.

Managing stress

Stress is part of all our lives and a bit of stress can motivate and drive people and provide meaningful challenges. Too much stress can trigger episodes of bipolar disorder. The aim of stress management is therefore not to eliminate stress, but to reduce it so that it does not have harmful effects. Some people seek ways of escaping that have long-term negative consequences, such as trying to drown their stress with alcohol. A number of more constructive strategies can provide relief from stress so that you can recharge your batteries, deal with the situation and prevent a build-up of stress. This can be even more effective if it becomes part of your routine; for example, scheduling a regular lunch with a friend whose company you find relaxing. Stress-relief strategies may also be useful when you encounter particularly difficult situations or major stressful events (see chapter 9). What works as a way to relieve stress differs from person to person. Here are some recommended ways of reducing stress:

Problem solving
Developing a problem-solving approach for confronting difficulties can make you feel much less overwhelmed and provides a constructive way forward. Sometimes when people are stressed or have symptoms of depression they tend to think negatively and blow minor difficulties into gigantic problems. It can be helpful to challenge your negative thinking, to regain your perspective before attempting to solve problems. Postponing problem solving if you are experiencing warning symptoms or an episode is a good idea, as you can focus on getting well and know that you will deal with problems later. When you are well, it might be easier to take your time to consider different solutions. Some simple problem-solving steps are provided on the website associated with this book, and an explanation and example of using problem solving to reduce interpersonal stress appears in chapter 19.

Taking time out
Part of reducing stress is about balancing activities that relieve stress with those things that provide stimulation and challenge, for example, watching sport on TV after you have spent hours

preparing an important presentation. You may also find that after taking a break you feel refreshed and can see things differently. Doing something enjoyable can lift your spirits when you feel stressed.

Supporting yourself

Sometimes people are so busy looking after everyone else that they don't take care of themselves. Acknowledging that things are tough, and being kind and gentle to yourself, can help in getting through a difficult situation. If you find your day has been filled with difficult things, give yourself a little treat. Activities which involve using the five senses—smell, touch, sight, hearing and taste—can be soothing (Linehan, 1993). You could listen to your favourite music, wear something that feels nice against your skin, enjoy the scent of flowers in your garden.

Supporting yourself also involves acting in your long-term interests. Examples include getting out of bed when you do not feel like it, reducing the amount of alcoholic drinks you consume, or coming home a bit earlier from a party to try to keep well.

Support from others

Being able to share your problem with a friend or a clinician can be helpful in reducing stress. There are many telephone help lines where you can talk to someone about your difficulties. Even just being with a friend whose company you find relaxing can help you to unwind.

Self-expression

Expressing feelings and thoughts through writing (such as in a journal) or by other means such as painting, sculpture, poetry or music, can help calm distressing thoughts and feelings and limit their ability to dominate your life.

Deep relaxation

Relaxation refers to the state of the body when stress and anxiety have been reduced. Specific bodily changes that occur during relaxation include decreases in heart rate, muscle tension, respiration rate and blood pressure. This is the opposite of what happens to our bodies during times of stress and anxiety. It is useful to practise relaxation techniques daily, as this will enable you to use relaxation at high-stress times as well as being a way of keeping day-to-day stress low.

Different people prefer different styles of relaxation. It can be worth persisting and trying a number of types to find one that works best for you. Types of relaxation include:

- *Breathing relaxation*, which uses a specific breathing technique that slows the heart rate and rate of breathing to achieve a feeling of relaxation.
- *Progressive muscular relaxation* or *Jacobson's relaxation*, which involves tensing and relaxing various muscle groups to create an awareness of where tension in the body accumulates and develop awareness of the difference between muscle tension and relaxation.
- *Autogenic relaxation*, which targets the autonomic nervous system, for example imagining warmth and increased blood flow to an area of the body to stimulate blood vessel dilation.
- *Imagery* or *visualisation relaxation*, which asks you to create an image of a calming, restful place or situation. This provides a distraction from stresses and evokes a relaxation response through the peaceful images. When practised routinely these images can be used in times of stress to help calm you.

When learning relaxation it is useful to choose a place where there will be minimal disruption, lie on your back, close your eyes and listen to a tape with a script instructing you what to do to relax. There are relaxation exercises in the resources mentioned on the website attached to this book.

Say 'no' wisely

Sometimes people find it hard to acknowledge that they have a right to protect their health, and to say no to excessively demanding things that may make them feel stressed and affect mood. This does not mean saying no to every demand, for then you will be going to the opposite extreme of over-protecting yourself and miss potential opportunities to participate in life. Saying no to things that are enticing but overstimulating is also necessary sometimes, such as being selective when you have a number of social invitations in the same week and do not want to disrupt your body clock.

Get organised

If there are many demands in a situation, making a list of priorities and dividing them into smaller steps, or postponing and delegating things, can make you feel less stressed. Set a timeframe for what can be realistically achieved. Tell yourself that you can only do what you can do in that situation and timeframe.

Choices

Being mindful of your choices in a stressful situation that is difficult to change can help you to feel less stuck. Leaving a stressful work environment might be the right option, but you can accept things the way they are if there is no way of changing them and you don't want to leave. For example, Gary loved his part-time job although one of his colleagues was very difficult to work with, and occasionally made things really stressful. He tried to sort out the problem but it became clear things were not likely to change. He decided to stay in the situation, and to develop strategies for dealing with this person when he became difficult. This kind of acceptance is about taking an active stand to use specific strategies to make the most of how things are. It does not mean that you will not decide to change the situation should this become possible.

When dealing with a difficult situation, whether or not you decide to stay or go, you can choose to make things worthwhile, to create pleasurable experiences and meaning and to take time out and reduce the stress.

Step by step

If you are in a difficult situation that is not readily changeable, taking things one step at a time and setting small achievable goals can make things easier. Remind yourself that it will not always be this way. Things in life rarely stay the same, even if you cannot directly change them. As life moves on, you never know what may happen to change a difficult situation down the track.

The pain and pleasure

Feelings are neither good nor bad in themselves. They are bodily reactions that give colour to our lives. As much as we all wish otherwise, painful and unpleasant feelings occur in life. The joy that occurs when we love, the hurt when we are let down, the shame when we have made mistakes, and the anger when we are treated unfairly, relate to specific situations at a specific time. They are not the whole of life, nor will the feelings, good or bad, remain at that intensity for all time. Using mindfulness techniques, where you are mindful of your thoughts and feelings without being drawn into them, may help to reduce stress (Segal et al., 2002).

Spiritual relief

For some people, prayer or getting in touch with their spiritual adviser helps relieve stress.

Healthy diet

Dietary guidelines suggest that we have foods from the five major food groups every day. These include breads and cereals; fruit; vegetables; meat, fish and poultry; and milk or milk products. A dietician can provide valuable assistance in establishing healthy eating habits. Having regular meal times is part of maintaining a regular routine and helps people keep to dietary changes. A healthy diet can help you to stay free of the burden of additional physical illnesses and obesity. 'Eating right should not be regarded as a cure for a mood disorder, but common sense dictates that what works for the heart and other organs also applies to the brain' (McManamy, 2006:155).

Research into the relationship between mood and diet is only starting to be done. Nevertheless, a diet high in omega-3 fatty acids derived largely from seafood is considered useful (Sontrop & Campbell, 2006). There is also evidence that folic acid, found in green leafy vegetables, may be helpful to some people, particularly with depression that resists treatment (Abou-Saleh & Coppen, 2006). Vitamin D, which is mainly made in the skin from sun exposure, is commonly deficient in Western populations. Supplementation may be useful for depression (Dumville et al., 2006). Many people report the benefits of eating healthy foods and cutting down on junk food, sugar, alcohol and caffeine.

Avoid toxic substances

Caffeine can interfere with your sleep, make you more anxious and agitated, restless and overactive, so if these are vulnerable areas for you, it might be important to consider alternatives. As we saw in earlier chapters, excessive alcohol and taking street drugs can trigger episodes of bipolar disorder. Smoking is not good for your health in general, and can contribute to your bipolar illness too. Smokers have more bipolar symptoms than non-smokers and may be less likely to respond to treatment. Attempting to stop smoking may help you stay well.

KEY POINTS

- There is no perfect lifestyle. You can choose to do things that help you to keep well and enjoy life.
- There may be times when you are symptomatic and need to focus on getting well and other times when you can participate in the richness of life, while keeping an eye on your bipolar disorder. Taking stabilising medications and maintaining

regular sleep and activity patterns are some of the ways of attending to your health when you are well.

- Participating in life and having social contact and relating to others can restore your sense of enjoyment and purpose. You can set realistic goals around the things that are important to you and pursue them in a way that does not trigger your bipolar symptoms. Doing things that make you feel alive and are in accordance with your strengths, abilities and talents and that do not interfere with your health can be healing.

- Other good habits, such as exercise, stress management, a healthy diet and avoiding toxic substances, can become part of a healthy lifestyle.

19 MAINTAINING CLOSE RELATIONSHIPS

Shared joy is a double joy; shared sorrow is half a sorrow.
Swedish proverb

Supportive relationships help people to enjoy life, deal with stress and get things done. They have been found repeatedly to have emotional and physical health benefits, and this is also true for bipolar disorder, where supportive relationships can help reduce the risk of relapse (Johnson et al., 1999; Johnson et al., 2003). On the other hand, criticism, hostility or overinvolvement and over-protectiveness can become destructive patterns that increase the risk of relapse (Miklowitz et al., 1988).

Support that enhances self-esteem is particularly helpful in reducing depressive relapse (Johnson et al., 2000). Respect and positive feedback that encourages a person's competence, rather than trying to take over, is good for your health and for your relationship. Support that is reciprocated, even in little ways, can keep a relationship alive. Doing enjoyable things together and sharing experiences also enrich a relationship.

In any relationship, people will have concerns and disagreements from time to time. This chapter explores some strategies for dealing with disagreements and criticism, and preserving and enhancing relationships with family and friends. Some of these strategies are derived from family-focused therapy, a therapy approach that has been shown to help reduce relapse in bipolar disorder (Miklowitz et al., 2003). More detail about these strategies can be found in Miklowitz's book *The Bipolar Disorder Survival Guide*. If you are experiencing serious difficulties in your relationship, we recommend involving a trained family or relationship counsellor to contribute a more objective perspective. Sometimes, of course, a relationship does not weather the storms, and we present some ideas for ways of managing when relationships end.

THINGS TO KEEP IN MIND

Symptoms of bipolar illness can temporarily influence the way you communicate with relatives and friends, thus it is preferable to deal with relationship concerns and conflict when you are feeling better. If either you or a loved one is too upset or angry to sort things out effectively, or become upset or angry when trying to do so, it is better to postpone discussions until you are both a bit calmer. If tempers flare every time you try to sort out the problem, get professional assistance.

COMMUNICATION SKILLS

Giving positive feedback, communicating about symptoms, active listening and making positive requests can reduce destructive ways of relating and promote good relationships.

Positive feedback

While it is important to communicate our concerns and sort out disagreements, it is also important to communicate our appreciation and recognition when someone does something we like. Positive feedback can encourage self-esteem, build mutual respect and a way of relating that acknowledges individual qualities and contributions. People are more likely to continue doing things if they receive positive feedback. Saying something like 'I can see you are making an effort to keep the house tidy, and I really appreciate it' may reinforce this behaviour. It can also provide a strong foundation for dealing with concerns.

Communicating about symptoms

Not all relationship problems for people with bipolar disorder are connected to the disorder, and it can be unhelpful to attribute every difficulty to it. Sometimes, however, a major cause of relationship problems is that relatives and friends lack information or misinterpret symptoms as being part of your personality, or a real reflection of how you feel about your relationship. For example, manic symptoms such as spending sprees, promiscuity and aggression may be misinterpreted as deliberate and controllable rather than understood as symptoms of illness. Information about your typical symptoms before, during and after an episode and the biological causes of bipolar disorder, and what helps, can assist those close to you in dealing with episodes. Recognising symptoms may prevent both you and your loved ones from pursuing conversations where it is not you but rather the bipolar disorder talking. Such 'bipolar conversations' (Fast & Preston, 2004) often lead to unnecessary conflict.

> Everything she did just irritated me. The way she served the same old dinner. The way she let the kids mess all over the house. How slow she was to understand all these great ideas I had been having. I found reasons to argue about everything and then suddenly she started to cry. I put the pieces together and realised that I was becoming manic. I knew I had to tell her about why I was so irritable, before it was too late. **Ned**

Providing information

How much detail to go into when providing information about your illness, or explaining it, always depends on the nature of the relationship—for example, a friend may not need to know as much as a partner or parent. It may be appropriate to discuss how important it is to you and your relationship for the other person to know a bit about the illness, and to encourage questions and discussions. Some people find it helpful to invite a close relative to accompany them to a doctor's appointment or support group to find out more about bipolar disorder and its management. It can be vital to convey that you are suffering from a treatable illness and not a character flaw.

If your loved ones want to be involved in this aspect of your life, being able to communicate how you experience symptoms, the warning signs and what you think triggers your illness, as well as the rationale behind treatments and lifestyle changes, can be an important step to involving them as allies in your plans to prevent or reduce relapse. The next step is negotiating ways they can help that suit both you and them.

When you notice symptoms

Telling those you love that you are developing particular symptoms can pre-empt damage to relationships. This is not always easy when you are symptomatic, and sometimes you might not realise that you have symptoms, but if you do, it can be helpful to communicate your insight.

When they notice symptoms

Many people with bipolar disorder find inaccurate assumptions that they are ill to be hurtful and disempowering. You and those close to you may be able to find a mutually acceptable way of their checking out whether a change they have noticed in you is indeed a symptom of illness. This clarification can prevent confusion and misinterpretation of symptoms, and also help you to catch symptoms early and reduce relapse. It can help to discuss your typical warning and actual symptoms with key people when you are well, and to include how you would like them to approach you if they notice any of these symptoms. Timing is important when discussing sensitive symptoms—an important tip for your relatives and friends is to communicate their genuine concern and/or confusion rather than to accuse or label you.

When people are symptomatic they might temporarily lose their usual insight into their behaviour. This can be the case particularly in a manic or mixed episode, and at that point it can be far wiser for relatives and friends to act to get professional help than to argue about symptoms.

Active listening

All too often people do not take the time to really listen to each other, to try to see the other's point of view. If they did, there would be far fewer misunderstandings, and meaningful compromises could be more easily reached. Active listening is about being able to see how you are both contributing to the problem so that you can sort it out.

Difficulties in relationships are easier to tackle if you understand where the other person is coming from.

Active listening is about doing the listening instead of the talking, about not giving your opinion immediately. It is not just hearing. It is really listening and asking for clarification by paraphrasing what you have heard, until you understand how the other person sees things. This means that there is no blame, and that the listener does not express their side of the argument. Active listening involves:

- *contact*: making eye contact with the speaker
- *attention*: focusing your attention on what the other person is saying
- *acknowledgment*: acknowledging what you heard by nodding your head, indicating that you have heard them or asking them to continue

- *check out*: asking questions and repeating what you have heard to check that you have understood their point of view. This will also help the other person to realise that you really have understood what they are saying.

Some people find it useful to take a moment once they have actively listened to another to reflect on what they have heard, see what their own needs are, and what they would like to see change. This is a useful first step to making a positive request and sorting out problems.

Positive requests

Making positive requests can be helpful when you need to be assertive, or to sort out conflicts. This technique involves specific and detailed communication, not about what the other person has done wrong, but rather what you would like to see change. Although sometimes you might need to do this on your own, it can be useful if both people in a relationship participate in this type of communication. When people are clear and direct about their needs there is less chance of miscommunication. Making positive requests involves:

- facing the person and making eye contact
- using 'I' statements—for example, 'I would like your help with . . .'
- telling them what you would like them to do. Be specific and avoid asking for many things at once. Make requests, not demands or commands. Don't apologise for your request, and avoid undercurrents of blaming. Try not to criticise; rather, focus on positive change. This works best if done in a calm and collected manner, without emotional heat.
- include how you think this could benefit you and where possible, the other person.

Here are some examples of making positive requests:

- 'I would like you to call me if you are going to come home late from work so I can prepare dinner later, and avoid being uptight about it being spoilt. Then we can have a nice quiet dinner together.'
- Making positive requests is a way of using the understanding you have gained from active listening to deal assertively with a situation. Sid had recently recovered from an episode of bipolar depression. Although he was much better, he still felt a bit lethargic and withdrawn so was still doing much less around the house than usual. Jessie, his partner, complained that he was being lazy and selfish. After Sid actively listened to Jessie, he realised that she felt that she relied on him, and found it hard to cope when he was depressed. He requested, 'I understand that you are very tired after the stress of my depressive episode, but it hurts me when you accuse me of having flaws that are actually symptoms left over from my depression. I would like you to find out more about my depression and residual symptoms, so you know that I am not to blame. Then we can discuss ways of making these times easier for both of us.' Jessie agreed and explained that she felt bad as she really knew that he was still not his usual self, and it would be good to find out more and have some practical strategies for dealing with these times together.

If someone does not agree to your positive request

Others may not agree to your positive requests. In some situations, difficulties in finding an agreement when making positive requests provide clues to more deep-seated problems that will require further problem solving or negotiation.

SORTING OUT PROBLEMS

Problem solving is a helpful way of dealing with interpersonal difficulties.

It is a way of stepping back and taking control of stressful situations. At certain times in every relationship there will be arguments and difficulties, and it can be useful to problem solve around these issues and sort them out. Not all problems are related to bipolar disorder. Practical problems can arise over financial issues, daily demands, child rearing, social plans, and ways of managing symptoms and their consequences. Sometimes more serious patterns, of emotional or sexual withdrawal, indifference, criticism, hostility, frequent arguments or over-protectiveness develop. People have found the problem-solving steps below helpful in dealing with both practical everyday problems and the more severe kinds.

How do you problem solve?

Some problems are easily solved, but other more difficult ones take greater time and effort. Problem solving is about trying out solutions and seeing what works. There is no passing or failing. Part of the solution may lie in enlisting the support of a neutral and skilled professional, ideally someone who has been trained in family or couple therapy.

When there are a number of problems, it can be necessary to prioritise them and work on one at a time. You can use the various communication skills discussed above to clarify what the problem is and to negotiate solutions.

Ideally, it is most effective to problem solve together with the other person or people in the relationship, but sometimes they may be unavailable or unwilling, and you will need to proceed on your own. If you change your behaviour towards your relative or close friend by using active listening, positive requests and problem solving, even if they are not responsive at first, in time they may become more receptive to this way of communicating (Miklowitz, 2002). In addition, rewarding any efforts on their part to improve things may further encourage this behaviour.

Tessa and her parents use problem-solving steps

Tessa was a 20-year-old university student, living with her parents, when she had her second manic episode. It took time to recover from the psychotic mania, but she did well in her journalism course. Although her mood stabilised nine months ago, her parents insisted on accompanying her to the doctor, and sometimes she felt that she might as well not have been in the room, because they did most of the talking. Tessa was becoming angry with her parents; she felt that they were being intrusive and overprotective, and her relationship with them was deteriorating. Her parents were worried that she might relapse and were trying to prevent this happening. They all made a conscious decision to use active listening to try to understand each other's point of view and to make positive requests to help sort out the problem (see figure 19.1).

Different solutions for different situations

There are no magical solutions that can be applied to all problems. For example, unlike Tessa, Sid (see earlier example) found that once Jessie began to understand his bipolar disorder, he liked her to accompany him to the doctor from time to time. Other couples may feel differently. Using relationship skills can help you find what works for you.

WORKABLE COMPROMISES

The following additional tips can help you reach a workable compromise when you have made your request or tried to problem solve, but the other person has an opposing viewpoint or cannot agree on a solution:

- Discuss trying to reach a win-win solution whereby both you and the other person benefit so that the outcome is fair to both of you.

Figure 19.1 Tessa's problem-solving steps

---

1. What is the problem?

(*Be as specific as possible and see whether you need to break the problem into a number of related problems. Prioritise which problem to tackle first.*)

- Tessa thinks her parents take over when they accompany her to her doctor's appointment, and she wants to attend on her own as part of taking charge of managing her illness. However, her parents feel it is important they attend the appointments as a way of helping to prevent relapse.
- This problem relates to the broader problem of Tessa needing more independence in terms of the management of her illness, but it is necessary to deal with the specific immediate issue first.

2. Brainstorm possible solutions

(*Think of as many as you can.*)

1. Tessa attends her doctor's appointments on her own.
2. Tessa's parents accompany her but let Tessa do the talking. Her parents could sit in on some of the appointment only.
3. Tessa attends the appointments on her own but keeps her parents up to date about her treatment, for example, her lithium levels and changes to her medications.
4. Her parents do not attend regularly, but can request to be included in an appointment with her doctor if they have any concerns about her treatment, or think she has warning signs of illness.
5. They discuss this problem with the doctor.

3. Evaluate all possible solutions

(*What are the steps in carrying out each solution? Is the solution practical? What resources do you need? What are the risks and consequences of each solution, and the advantages vs. disadvantages?*)

continued

They weighed up the advantages and disadvantages of each solution and what steps might be involved in the solutions. For example, solution 1 increased Tessa's parents' anxiety whereas solution 2 made her feel that she still could not discuss things with her doctor independently. They all liked solutions 3 and 4, which gave Tessa more independence but let her feel that they were there to support her.

4. Select your solution(s)

They decided that Tessa would attend her doctor's appointments on her own and would give them feedback about her treatment, and that they could ask to accompany her to the doctor if they had concerns or noticed warning signs of illness. If this did not work out they decided they would try solution 5, discussing things with the doctor.

5. Plan the solution

(*What resources will you need? What time frame? What might you need to do first?*)

They agreed that Tessa would attend her next doctor's appointment on her own and that she would give her parents feedback and keep them informed about her lithium levels or any side effects she was experiencing. Her parents told her that they would tell her if they were concerned about her treatment or if they noticed signs of illness and wanted to accompany her to the doctor. Tessa said she would explain the solutions they were trying to her doctor.

6. Implement the plan

(*This involves putting the plan into practice.*)

They implemented the plan.

7. Did it work?

(*Assess whether your solution(s) have been helpful, and return to step 2 if you need to adjust the solution or find a new one.*)

continued

The solution regarding the doctor's appointment worked well for all of them. Tessa's parents developed a new respect for their daughter's independence in managing her illness, which spilled over into her life, and their relationship improved. Tessa felt that they have grown closer through learning how to let go a bit.

8. Encourage yourselves
(*Working on problems is not easy, and all efforts deserve to be acknowledged. Not all problems have immediate solutions, and finding what works for you can take time.*)
Tessa told her parents how much she values their belief in her and the way they have her interests at heart. Her parents explained that they admire her for the way she has dealt with all of this.

- Brainstorm the alternatives and make a list to see what is acceptable to both parties.
- If this is not possible and the person does not want to give you what you want, ask for a counterproposal. If you do not like this proposal, you give a counterproposal and so on.
- Ask, 'What do you need from me to be able to do this my way?' Possibilities include, 'My way this time, your way next time'; 'Meet me halfway'; 'If you do this for me, I'll do that for you'; 'My way when I am doing it and your way when you are'.
- Agree to differ. Even people in a good relationship agree to differ about certain issues.

ENJOYING YOUR RELATIONSHIP

Enjoying 'bipolar-free time' together and regaining intimacy can reinforce relationships.

Enjoying 'bipolar-free time' together

Attending to your health and sorting out conflicts and problems in your relationship are important, but enjoying time together and sharing interests and responsibilities can strengthen the bond and sustain it through hard times. Julie Fast and John Preston, in their book *Loving Someone with Bipolar Disorder* (2004), advocate the healing power of laughing together and having time together in a 'bipolar-free zone'.

Regaining emotional and sexual intimacy

Low libido is a symptom of depression, and your sexual relationship may recover spontaneously when the depression lifts. Sometimes emotional and sexual intimacy between partners deteriorates due to the strain of living with bipolar disorder, and people find that they need time to get to know each other again after an episode of illness. It helps if your partner has some understanding of bipolar disorder and a positive attitude about its management. Good communication and problem solving can help sort out conflicts and prevent resentment and anger from building up. Doing enjoyable activities together can help build up your friendship again and make it easier to restore sexual intimacy.

Taking things slowly, not putting yourself or your partner under too much pressure, and focusing on relaxed sexual enjoyment is recommended. Not having too high expectations, and persisting when sexual intimacy does not come as easily as before, can also be helpful. In some situations, it can be useful to enlist the help of a sex therapist, who may give you a program to follow at home to gradually rekindle your sexual relationship.

CURBING CRITICISM

Some people are particularly sensitive to criticism. If you (or your partner or other loved ones) fall into this category, remember there are other ways of expressing concern or dissatisfaction. Good communication skills and problem solving can reduce the problem. For example, instead of blaming someone for being untidy, you can positively request that they join you in brainstorming how to keep the place tidier, because that might help you to feel less irritable; this might mean getting more cupboard space or developing a joint tidy-up time before watching TV together. If criticism has become a pattern in your relationship, you may need to enlist professional counselling.

Ideas for dealing with criticism include:

Good communication

In any close relationship it is not surprising to have concerns about each other, but these concerns need to be expressed and addressed constructively, and balanced with positive feedback about good behaviour. It is important that concerns about a person's behaviour are expressed as concerns about their behaviour, rather than attacks on who they are as a person. It is more useful to focus on positive requests for future change, rather than to focus on blaming a person for their past behaviour.

If someone is criticising you, you can use active listening and check that what you hear them saying is what they actually mean. This alone can sometimes make the other person soften so you are able to clarify your point of view and discuss their concerns more amicably. You can make a positive request that they change the way they are expressing their concern if they are being very negative and blaming, and ask them to paraphrase their concern in a more constructive way indicating specifically what they would like to see change (perhaps a bit later when feelings have calmed down). It may also be useful to give those close to you information on active listening and making positive requests, and to discuss how you can change the way concerns are expressed in your relationship. Family therapy helps people get used to expressing concerns in a more positive way and to respond to these concerns constructively.

Do not jump to conclusions

When you are feeling particularly sensitive or have symptoms of depression you may sometimes interpret a remark as criticism when it is not. It can be worth using the Helpful Thought Summary (see chapter 12) to see whether you have jumped to the wrong conclusion.

Distance yourself

There are many reasons why a person may feel critical. Daily life can be filled with stress, and people often tend to take this out on each other. Sometimes a person feels overwhelmed, or does not understand all the different aspects of a situation, and blaming you (or you blaming them) may be a way of trying to make sense of things. Criticism is sometimes used in defence when a person believes that they are being challenged or undermined. It may be used impulsively when they feel irritable. This style of communication sometimes says more about the person who is being critical than about the person who is the object of the attack. Although it is hard if you are on the receiving end, putting some distance between yourself and the criticism, and asking yourself why the other person is resorting to it, can help you to understand and address the problem. It may be a little easier if you are able to see the criticism in context and do not just take it at face value.

Make it constructive

Even if the criticism was meant to be malicious, if there is a grain of truth in it you can remind yourself that no one is perfect and use this understanding to your advantage.

COPING IF THE RELATIONSHIP ENDS

In some relationships, things deteriorate so far and become so destructive that the best solution may be to go your separate ways. It is best to make such weighty decisions when you are well. As Rhonda says, 'Be selective. Stay away from people who are toxic to your mood. Choose which relationships you want to work at and which are too damaging.'

There are different ways of ending a relationship. One is a slow transformation culminating in less contact, but there can also be a more abrupt and sharper parting of ways. There is always pain involved when you have been close to someone, but it can be helpful to prepare yourself if you are certain the relationship is going to end. You can do this by involving yourself in more activities without that person, rebuilding other social relationships and pursuing other interests. It is normal to grieve if you have lost a relationship, and to feel a range of emotions such as sadness, anger, guilt or relief. Many people find it beneficial to talk to their clinician or a grief counsellor about their feelings. It can also help to take things day by day, to try to continue your usual routine, and to plan some distracting and soothing activities. The way the relationship ends can make a difference, and it is worth trying to end it as amicably as possible to prevent even more heartache.

KEY POINTS
- Although not all problems in relationships are caused by bipolar disorder, this illness can put a strain on important relationships.
- Good relationships not only enrich life but also may help protect you from relapse.
- You and those you care about can do a lot to maintain close relationships and allow them to grow, including:
  - giving positive feedback
  - helping those who matter to understand about the illness, and finding ways to communicate with each other about symptoms
  - using active listening and making positive requests
  - problem solving and trying out different solutions
  - finding workable compromises
  - focusing on enjoying bipolar-free time and rebuilding the relationship

- finding ways to enhance the positive expression of concerns and to reduce criticism and its distressing effect on you
- getting professional help from a relationship, family or sex therapist.
- Sometimes a relationship becomes too destructive and it must end. You may need time to grieve, and input from your support network.

20 YOU AND YOUR DOCTOR

I flailed against the sentence I felt he had handed me. He listened to my convoluted, alternative explanations ... He was very tough, as well as very kind, and even though he understood more than anyone how much I was losing—in energy and vivacity, and originality—by taking medication, he never was seduced into losing sight of the overall perspective of how costly, damaging, and life-threatening my illness was ... He treated me with respect, a decisive professionalism, wit, and an unshakable belief in my ability to get well, compete and make a difference.

Kay Jamison, *An Unquiet Mind*, 1997:87.

People with bipolar disorder can sometimes feel very alone and confused about dealing with their illness. Having someone who is knowledgeable about treatment options and who can understand things from your perspective can be an enormous relief. Having a good relationship with your doctor is an important factor in the treatment of bipolar disorder. The US National Depressive and Manic-Depressive Association survey in 2000 (Hirschfeld et al., 2003) found that those who were more satisfied with their doctor were better able to come to terms with their illness, felt better able to cope with the illness and were less ashamed or angry about it. But what constitutes a 'good' doctor–patient relationship? You might have your personal preferences about things that are important in your relationship with your doctor. There is no single defining element of a good doctor–patient relationship; rather, a number of related elements are involved.

LEVEL OF COLLABORATION

Historically, the relationship between doctor and patient has been a directive one, in which the doctor takes the lead and advises the patient on what to do. More recent times, however, have seen a trend towards a more collaborative relationship between doctor and patient, a relationship in which both parties contribute and work towards the effective management of the illness.

People differ in which approach they find most suitable for them. Many people enjoy collaborating with their doctors:

My doctor always explains about different treatments and side effects, and I can ask him anything. He knows that I will monitor things and give him feedback about how things are going. We discuss different medication options and make decisions together. **Madeleine**

The appropriateness of the more directive style compared with a more collaborative style will also vary according to the phase of the illness (Berk et al., 2004). If you are very unwell, for example, your doctor might need to temporarily assume a more directive role and admit you to hospital. This may be part of your own relapse prevention plan.

A COLLABORATIVE APPROACH

A number of things help to form a strong collaborative alliance between doctor and patient: communication, trust, reliability, continuity, caring and respect. This alliance also makes it easier at times when your doctor needs to play a more directive role in your treatment.

Communication

A collaborative relationship involves a partnership between you and your doctor whereby each person values and respects the other's contribution. Your doctor may be an expert on medication, but you are the expert on your experience of your illness. Monitoring your moods and the effects of your treatment gives you an advantage when communicating with your doctor. Together you make a team.

Asking questions and being ready to voice concerns is a way of getting the most from your treatment. This includes talking about your symptoms as well as the things that go well, and about the difficulties, such as possible side effects of medication. People have a range of different views about medication. Discussing your rationale for wanting to take or not take medication, and what you are hoping to get out of treatment, can help the doctor to understand your needs. In return, the doctor might be able to provide you with alternative options and updated information, so that you can make more informed decisions about treatment.

Honest communication between you and the doctor means treatment options can be openly considered. As one psychiatrist commented, 'I would much rather a patient tell me if they hadn't followed through on what was planned. That way we can discuss other options together so that they can get the best results from treatment.' Not raising your concerns can also cause you additional stress and worry.

Knowing that your doctor is not judging you, sincerely has your interests at heart and will express an honest view about your treatment can make open communication much easier. When you are faced with a number of treatment options, it can be helpful to ask your doctor, based on their knowledge, what they consider the best option to be.

While for some people communication with doctors is exclusively related to symptoms and medication, others discuss other illness-management skills, such as regulating their sleep and activities, and dealing with relationships or stressful events. As part of this communication, it is the role of the doctor to provide information in a way that makes sense to you (that is, without excessive medical terminology). Written information that you can take home can also be helpful.

There may be times when your doctor asks very specific questions regarding your mood and your thoughts. It is important, for example, if you are feeling depressed, for your doctor to have some understanding of the depth of your depression. Questions about thoughts or plans for hurting yourself or others could be asked at this time. For those who never experience these sorts of thoughts, such questions can seem out of place, but for those who face such despair there can be an enormous sense of relief in being able to talk about their disturbing thoughts. Suicidal thoughts and plans are temporary but dangerous symptoms of illness; discussing them can make you feel less isolated, help you gain another perspective and prevent a tragedy. If you experience these thoughts and your doctor does not ask you about them, you need to reveal them.

Trust

It is easier to feel comfortable about asking questions if you trust your doctor. There is a real sense of reassurance in being able to trust your doctor's knowledge, skill and reliability, in knowing that this person will always act in your best interest. Trusting that your doctor will listen to what you have to say and respect your perspective without being dismissive makes it much easier to discuss your concerns. This does not necessarily mean that your doctor will agree with you, and developing such a degree of trust can take time. And at times, of course, it can be difficult to 'hear' if your doctor is telling you that you are becoming unwell. As William says: 'I appreciate it when my doctor who knows me so well is honest if he thinks I am going high, even if it irritates me. I have learnt over time that he has my best interests at heart and so I consider what he says.'

There may be times when you are so severely ill that you need to trust your doctor to make temporary treatment decisions on your behalf, such as admitting you to a particular hospital. You can discuss these issues with your doctor when you are well as part of your plans to get more control over your illness.

Reliability

Reliability is also a shared element of a good doctor–patient relationship. It is important for your doctor to be reliable and to be trusted to be available or, when not available, to have a back-up that is acceptable to you in the event that warning signs or an episode occurs. It is also important for both you and your doctor to keep regularly scheduled appointments. Even if things are going well you should stick to agreements that have been made.

> A few times a year my doctor attends professional conferences, but he always makes sure I'm aware when he is going away if this is around my scheduled appointment time. He also provides the name of the doctor who will be covering his practice while he is away. I appreciate the fact that my doctor lets me know this. **James**

Continuity

Having regular appointments and building a strong relationship with the same doctor can mean that you get to know each other and build up trust more readily. Continuity can also come with a multidisciplinary team rather than an individual in some services.

You know what to expect from your doctor, and your doctor can gain a deeper understanding of your moods and what works for you, which can be a safety net when you become ill. Marianne says, 'I have been going to the same doctor for the past few years, and this has been an anchor for me through my turbulent moods, the ups and downs of relationships, moving house, and changing jobs.'

Caring and respect

You need to find a doctor whose knowledge and approach you can respect. Respect needs to be mutual. It is important to feel that your doctor cares about *you*, and is able to see you the person behind the illness. Remember that respecting another person's views does not mean that you have to always agree with them. Even if you and your doctor have some different views about things, if you know that your doctor is really committed to helping you manage your health in the long term and understands your struggle in managing the illness, you can develop a strong bond that can withstand differences of opinion.

There may be a time when you decide that you would like to enlist the help of an additional clinician, such as a psychologist, who has experience in bipolar disorder and who could help you with a particular aspect of your life, such as negative thoughts or anxiety. Letting your doctor know if you decide to see a psychologist means that you are all working as a coordinated team.

If you are struggling in working with your current doctor, or are not improving on your current treatment, getting a second opinion can be helpful. This is not something that you should be embarrassed about. Getting a second opinion is something that doctors frequently suggest, on their own initiative. Again, the important thing is that the doctors communicate, with any suggestions being fed back to your treating doctor rather than leaving you in the difficult position of having to decide between two potentially different opinions.

INVOLVING A SUPPORTIVE RELATIVE OR FRIEND

Many people with bipolar disorder, and the research evidence, support a collaborative approach to managing the illness that includes you, your loved ones and the clinician involved in your treatment. This does not mean that your doctor needs to break doctor–patient confidentiality or that you do not have control over the management of your illness. You can decide *if* you want your doctor to communicate with a particular relative or friend, and *what* you would like them to communicate. If you become very ill, you may need your close relative or friend to communicate with your doctor on your behalf and to help more actively with treatment.

> It was hard when my wife came along to my appointment with my doctor. Initially I felt a bit awkward, but it turned out to be beneficial. She has become part of the treatment team with my doctor, and she now has a better sense of my day-to-day struggles. This has strengthened our relationship. **Paul**

WHEN DIFFICULTIES ARISE

When difficulties arise in your relationship with your doctor, there are a number of things to consider.

* Try to identify the areas that you are not satisfied with and problem solve around them. For example, if you feel you do not get to spend enough time with your doctor, it might be worth discussing the possibility of booking a double appointment.
* If you have a difference in opinion regarding treatment, it is useful for both parties to really listen and understand the

other's point of view. It is also useful to get as much information on the topic as possible so you can weigh up the pros and cons and make a decision.

- Often people become annoyed with themselves when they leave their doctor's rooms and realise that they haven't talked about some of the things that have been concerning them. If this has happened to you, it can be useful to write things down before your appointment, take the list in with you and refer to it during the consultation.

- Sometimes doctors provide so much information that it seems overwhelming; it can be helpful to ask them to slow down or, if the information is too technical, to ask for an explanation. At the other extreme, sometimes a doctor may not provide enough information, and you need to ask for more.

- You may feel upset by some information your doctor has provided. It is important to mention that you feel upset, as this allows your doctor to explain a confusing issue, or suggest ways of looking at things that help put them in perspective.

- If you feel your doctor is not listening to what you say, this can be something you can raise directly; for example, 'I feel as if you have not really heard my concerns.' It can be particularly useful in this case to take someone you trust with you to the appointment.

- People report that having a GP who is knowledgeable and experienced in the treatment of bipolar disorder is also important. If there is no such doctor in your area it can be useful to enlist the cooperation of a psychiatrist who can advise your GP about treatment options.

- Remember you always have the right to get another opinion or find another doctor, but before you sever relationships with your current doctor, think about a few things:
  - Beware of making this decision if you are in an episode of illness, as you may not be thinking as clearly as you do when you are well.

- It can be useful to write down positive and negative things you find about the relationship and weigh them up. It could be that the positive outweighs the negative overall.
- You could try communicating your concerns and seeing if this brings about a positive change.
- Use the 48-hour rule and think about your decision before acting. Sometimes feelings of irritability can cloud the issue.
- Make sure you have another doctor to go to before cutting the relationship.
- Check that your expectations are realistic. It can sometimes take time to find the right treatment, even when your doctor is very knowledgeable and skilled.

KEY POINTS

- The importance of a good doctor–patient relationship is often underestimated. A good relationship with your doctor is not simply a nice thing to have; it can help you get the most from your treatment and stay well.
- A number of factors contribute to your relationship with your doctor. Some people prefer a more directive approach in their doctor–patient relationship, others prefer a more collaborative one. In bipolar disorder the phase of illness may influence the approach being taken.
- If you are experiencing difficulties in your relationship with your doctor, you can try and troubleshoot these problems.
- Good communication, trust, reliability, continuity, mutual caring and respect are aspects of a strong collaborative alliance between you and your doctor.

21 SOMEONE I CARE ABOUT HAS BIPOLAR DISORDER

What most people don't think of, is that a bipolar disorder diagnosis rocks more than one world.

Lori Oliwenstein, *Taming Bipolar Disorder*, 2004:319.

If you have a close relative or friend with bipolar disorder, this chapter is written for you. Bipolar disorder affects not only the life of the person with the illness, but also the lives of those who care about them, particularly if you are in frequent contact or living together.

Bipolar disorder, like any other illness, brings its own particular challenges which may be experienced quite differently by different people, depending on a number of factors. These include how ill the person is and how you both respond to the illness, as well as how you are related—whether you are a partner, parent, sibling, child or friend. Some family members report forming closer relationships with the person with bipolar disorder since receiving the diagnosis, others find their relationships more challenging (Dore & Romans, 2001; Michalak et al., 2006).

Relatives and close friends may find that their everyday life changes, and that at times they become exhausted and even depressed. There are ways of supporting your ill friend or relative in their battle with this chronic illness that can reduce the risk of relapse without sacrificing your own wellbeing. We discuss some of the changes that occur and ways of managing them in this chapter.

CHANGES IN EVERYDAY LIFE

Very little might change if your relative or friend is well most of the time. There may be some changes to your lifestyle if you are living with them, such as providing more structure and routine, or adapting to their strategies to prevent relapse. On the other hand, the changes may be extreme, and you can find that you reduce your work and corresponding income, as well as your social life, and neglect your own health, in order to look after the ill person.

Dealing with a loved one's bipolar disorder can cause significant stress (Dore & Romans, 2001). You are not alone if this is your experience. Supporting someone with bipolar disorder can be an isolating experience, especially if you do not have a good back-up system, such as access to supportive clinicians involved in their treatment and other people to help in specific ways when they are ill. More distress has been reported by relatives in situations where the ill person has had an episode within the previous two years, has rapid cycling, and where they are actively involved in the management of medications to treat the bipolar disorder. Your stress levels are influenced not only by the severity of the illness, but also by how much the illness interferes with daily life and how both you and the ill person cope (Reinares et al., 2006).

These changes can affect your relationship. Partners sometimes comment that when their loved one has been ill for a while and they have had to assume an almost parental role, they become emotionally and physically withdrawn. Some parents, on the other hand, report feeling closer to their ill children when they take a more active role in helping them to get well.

Symptoms such as withdrawal, irritability, anger and hyper-activity can put a strain on close relationships, while sexual relationships can suffer due to loss of libido due to depression or as a side effect of some medications. The deep fear when your loved one is suicidal is something many people face. Some of the consequences of manic behaviour, such as spending sprees and sexual exploits, can be stressful for all involved. Symptoms of bipolar disorder can sometimes mean that the person you know so well behaves in strange, unpredictable and disturbing ways, that the person you knew so well seems to have 'disappeared'. It can take time to recover your closeness and to find ways of dealing with bipolar disorder. Some people report that through this process they get to know themselves and their relative or friend better, and their relationship deepens.

UNDERSTANDABLE REACTIONS

You may find that your friend or relative's bipolar disorder is quite manageable, that you have both worked out ways of coping, and it is not difficult to enjoy life and time together. Some people find that they go through a period of grief as they try to come to terms with the illness, or that the stress of numerous demands results in a build-up of anger and emotional overload.

Grief

Just as the person with bipolar disorder may grieve for all those things that might have been if they did not have this illness, you also may go through times of shock, denial, sadness, anger, relief and acceptance. Grief can be experienced at other times, such as when a loved one relapses, but it is often particularly intense when they have recently been diagnosed and you are concerned about how the illness can be managed or what it means for the future. It can make a difference to find out more, speak to professionals and people who live well with bipolar disorder, and read about their experiences.

Build-up of anger

In any close relationship, anger can build up due to unmet needs and expectations, and the burden of extra demands due to illness can fuel the anger. In turn your loved one may feel that you are being undermining or overprotective, or don't really understand, or are being withdrawn and rejecting. If this anger is not channelled into communication to sort out the problems, into battling the illness rather than the person, and into taking time out for your own needs, it can threaten the relationship and increase stress for both of you. In every relationship, people have disagreements from time to time, but if disagreement is becoming the norm in your situation it may be time to take action to sort things out, possibly enlisting professional help.

Emotional overload

There may be times when you feel as if you are in emotional overload. This may involve sustained periods of feeling overwhelmed, flooded, too exhausted to think, very angry, anxious, depressed or burnt out, or being critical, hostile or overprotective towards your loved one. These are all signs that urgent attention needs to be given to your wellbeing as well, not just to the wellbeing of the person suffering from bipolar disorder. Emotional overload may be a message that it is time to explore new ways of coping and to seek professional help.

WHAT CAN HELP?

Every situation is personal and you need to find out what works for you. Here are some suggestions gathered from people who have experienced these changes, and from the literature, about what can make things easier.

Knowledge is power

General knowledge

Perhaps one of the most helpful things when someone you care about has bipolar disorder is to find out about the symptoms, the causes and treatments. Knowing what you are dealing with can make it much more manageable. This knowledge can be obtained from books, the Internet (see the resources section on www.randomhouse.co.uk/bipolar) and from professionals who work with people with bipolar disorder.

Specific knowledge

Another important type of knowledge is knowing about your loved one's particular experience of bipolar disorder—their symptoms, triggers, warning signs, and what works for them in managing their illness. Observing, and having discussions with your loved one when they are well, about what works in different phases of the illness can make it easier to provide appropriate support and lessen misunderstandings (see chapter 19).

Accepting bipolar disorder

Just as a person with bipolar disorder may react in various ways to their diagnosis, close friends and family members may respond to the illness by denying it, at the one extreme, or by becoming over-involved with it at the other. Many people find that acceptance of a loved one's bipolar disorder is the first step to adapting to it and making the most of things.

Denial of the illness

Denying the illness is sometimes a stage on the way to acceptance, and it is not uncommon for someone to return to this stage from time to time. Denial may be your way of protecting yourself or your loved one from some of the painful emotions that arise in facing the reality of this stigmatised diagnosis. You may believe that your ill relative or friend is 'stressed' or 'burnt out' and 'not crazy'. Denial can cause friction in your relationship because you may appear to be uninvolved while the person with bipolar disorder feels isolated and unsupported. You could find yourself criticising your relative or friend for not controlling behaviour that is actually part of the illness. Denial on your part could encourage them to ignore their illness and the need for treatment. Untreated bipolar disorder can be very disruptive.

Acceptance

Understanding that bipolar disorder is a recurrent illness and that there is a person behind the illness, as in any other illness, can help friends and relatives to accept the diagnosis and see beyond stig-matised labels. You may need to adapt your expectations to the reality of the situation and go through a period of grief over what you thought your lives or relationship would otherwise be like. Realising that there are helpful treatments and strategies for managing bipolar disorder can make it easier to accept.

Overinvolvement

Some people become overinvolved in their role as caregivers and feel the need to step in and take over even when their loved one is relatively well. This can undermine their ability to cope, and result in emotional overload for you. There may be times when the person is so ill that you do need to take a more active role, temporarily. On the other hand, there may be times when they are relatively well and letting go is supportive.

Emma was Neil's partner. He had experienced many episodes of mania but had not relapsed for two years and was working part time. Emma had read everything she could on the illness and took it upon herself to structure his life and see to his medications so that he would not relapse. Neil appreciated her devotion and concern but wished that she would trust him to see to his own medication and management strategies. He decided to let her know that he understood her concern and to explain how important it was for him to manage things more independently. Now that his illness was more under control he wanted to enjoy things with her and focus on their life together while he tried to keep well.

Rebecca Woolis, in *When Someone You Love has a Mental Illness*, advises, 'It is useful to keep two general principles in mind: first, let people do as much as they can for themselves; second, try to ensure that they feel your love and support' (Woolis, 2003:62).

You might expect that if a relative were very protective, involved and self-sacrificing in response to a loved one's bipolar disorder, the result would be good rates of adherence to prescribed medication regimes and better health outcomes. On the contrary, however, people whose caregivers tend to be overinvolved have poorer adherence to medication and are more likely to develop further episodes of illness (Perlick et al., 2004). This implies that a different approach to helping your loved one manage their illness may be necessary, which may involve accepting that different support is required in different phases of the illness. Wherever possible, supporting an individual's constructive coping strategies and autonomy in managing their illness may prove beneficial.

Maintaining healthy boundaries

Maintaining healthy boundaries between you and the ill person can relieve distress and prevent the build-up of anger. Things you can do to maintain healthy boundaries include:

- Acknowledge that you have feelings and needs, too.
- Prioritise if there are extra demands, and just focus on getting through one day at a time.
- Do not be scared to delegate to other willing family members or friends.

- Arrange time out. Do something nice for yourself.
- Devote even a little time to outside interests and try to keep up with your friends.
- Take care of your health.
- Remember that crises when your loved one is very symptomatic are temporary.
- Make sure you maintain a basic structure to your day and get enough to eat and enough sleep.
- Find someone to talk to whom you can trust or join a support group of like-minded people.
- Make use of online resources, especially if you are pressed for time.
- Try to see through the misconceptions involved in stigma.
- Keep in touch with your ill relative or friend's strengths.
- Be flexible in adapting your support to the situation—stand back when less active support is required, and have a plan of action when you need to take a more active role.
- Use communication skills to set clear limits about what you can and cannot do in different phases of the illness.
- Remember, it is not helpful to be overinvolved, and it is not *your* illness.
- Recognise that sometimes people need time and experience to learn the best ways of managing their illness, but set limits if their self-management becomes destructive.
- Accept that support can be reciprocated, and learn to receive support from your loved one and others.
- Don't expect to fix everything. No one can be 100 per cent in control of life all the time.
- Contact a therapist if you experience emotional overload.

Making plans

Although you cannot plan for every single eventuality, developing a written plan for yourself about your involvement and its limitations can make living with this challenging illness a little more predictable. Plans need to be flexible as sometimes the demands of the illness and treatments may change, and supportive people may come and go. It is important to learn from experience and adapt plans accordingly.

Ask how you can help

It is vital to let the ill person do as much as they can for themselves and not to undermine their competence. You could enquire if they could use any assistance in managing their illness and what they think might be helpful—for example, they might ask you to assist them in recognising warning signs, to call the doctor when they are too ill to do so themselves, or to contact their work to let them know they are ill. Your involvement might differ depending on whether you are a friend, partner, parent, child or sibling. Deciding what you cannot do is as important as deciding what you can do. You also need to consider your own wellbeing in drawing up these plans.

You might consider contributing to any of the following areas and discussing this with your relative or friend:

- Helping them to reduce their specific triggers of bipolar disorder and implement healthy lifestyle changes.
- Recognising and responding to warning symptoms.
- How to help if things get worse or when your relative or friend is recovering from an episode.
- Whether and in what circumstances your relative or friend wants you to play a role in contacting doctors or in supporting their medical treatment (for example, getting scripts filled, reminding them to take medication if they are very ill or making treatment decisions on their behalf).
- How your involvement with their illness needs to change when they are well.
- How to respond to crises—for example, if they are planning to do something with very risky consequences, are becoming aggressive, or have suicidal symptoms.

Good communication

To avoid miscommunication, you might need to clarify that you do not wish to take over the management of your loved one's illness, that you understand that they are in charge of it. Ideally, you may be able to develop your own management plan in conjunction with your loved one's relapse prevention and suicide risk management plans. Forming a team, with your relative or friend with bipolar disorder as captain, and which involves yourself and their clinician(s), provides the best chance of keeping bipolar disorder under control (Bauer & McBride, 2003).

You can plan on your own

If your relative or close friend is not keen to involve you in their plans to manage their illness, it may be possible to respect their wishes but still make plans in so far as the illness affects you. For example, you may work out a way of coping or lifestyle changes that are convenient for you. Even if your loved one does not want to collaborate, you can work out what you could do to protect both of you in a crisis, such as if they become suicidal. Your hopeful, non-judgmental and proactive approach may help them realise that there are other ways of dealing with bipolar disorder and that they do not have to manage it all alone.

Blame doesn't help

In an effort to make sense of a loved one's illness, it is natural to look for something to blame. Bipolar disorder is complex, with many possible causes and triggers, so attributing blame to yourself or others is a waste of time. People have found that accepting the complexity of the illness and having many strategies for dealing with it is much more helpful than blaming.

'It's my genes'

Parents sometimes blame themselves for passing on bipolar genes and suffer painful guilt. Stop here a minute—consider these questions: Even if you have passed on these bipolar genes, where did you get them from? Before that, where did your ancestors get them, and so on and so on? Also, remember that there are many pathways to bipolar disorder, that genetics is not the whole story.

Unrealistic expectations of yourself

Some people wish that they could be a better partner or friend, or find better ways to reduce stressful triggers. There are no perfect relatives or friends. Do you expect to be the perfect support, never criticise, never get angry, never try to control things, and never feel like running away? All these feelings are normal from time to time, and there are ways of coping constructively with this illness. Managing things on a day-by-day basis can help to get through the more difficult patches. Although things can look bleak, the illness often improves as people find new or different ways to manage it. Occasionally the situation may become so destructive to your wellbeing that you need to get help, or even leave. Coping well does *not* mean sacrificing yourself.

Unrealistic expectations of others

Sometimes it seems to make sense to blame the person with the bipolar disorder. It is all too easy to confuse symptoms with personality, and to blame the person for not having more control over their actions. This criticism may increase the chances of relapse and undermine your relationship.

> Sharon had bipolar II disorder and as she realised she was becoming ill, put her plan to reduce depression into place. Tony, her partner, accused her of being moody, irresponsible, and not even bothering to snap out of it. There was nothing he could say against her that she had not said herself. However, it was hard having this confirmed. It made her feel so guilty, so alone, and even more depressed.

Unrealistically high expectations of the sufferer's ability to control the illness can lead to harsh words when relapse occurs. Much can be done to keep well, but no one can control everything perfectly all the time, especially when it comes to a complex illness like bipolar disorder. Finding what works to best deal with illness can be a matter of trial and error. What works sometimes changes over time, and may be different in different situations. You might need to adjust your plans to cope with the illness. Sometimes, despite a person's best efforts to manage their illness, breakthrough episodes occur. Recognising your loved one's efforts to control their illness and to make the most of life can help build their self-esteem.

Another common time for unrealistic expectations is just after an episode. People need time to return to usual tasks and to deal with accumulated demands. Sometimes people need to make more permanent adjustments to their lifestyle due to their bipolar illness.

Disagreeing about ways of coping

If you think the way your relative or friend is managing their illness is not helpful, blame and resentment can build up. Ultimately, however, it is *their* illness, and they have the responsibility of deciding how to manage it. You can communicate your concern and invite discussion in positive ways without taking these decisions away from them and taking over, or becoming very critical. Jim actively listened to his son's reasons for wanting to throw away his medications and requested:

> I understand that you feel well and want no reminders of your episodes but I feel worried about you relapsing, especially around exam time. This has happened before, so I am not sure it is the best time to go off your medication. Maybe it would be an idea to discuss this decision with your doctor in case it jeopardises your exams and plans.

On the other hand, your loved one might routinely refuse responsibility for managing their illness or simply deny the need for treatment, or use self-destructive ways of coping, such as taking alcohol and drugs. This means that you are faced with untreated bipolar disorder, which can lead to emotional overload on both your parts. It can be helpful to try to reason with them if they are not too ill or intoxicated, and to point out the consequences (that you consider might matter to them), of continuing in this way. In addition, your positive requests for change could include explanations of the ways the illness is affecting you and your relationship. You could invite them to problem solve with you about how best you can both move forward, or accompany them to their clinician. As part of your own plan to deal with the illness, you could establish ground rules that include what you are prepared to tolerate—for example, that you are happy to take over their duties when they are ill if they agree to seek help for their drinking problem, which is making their bipolar disorder worse. If they refuse to change, you may need to protect yourself and limit your involvement.

It is not wise to threaten that you will leave or withdraw your support unless you have tried everything else, and unless you really mean it. Otherwise you lose credibility in your supportive role, and thus make the situation potentially more difficult. Getting professional help in these situations can make a big difference.

Things that will sustain you both

Besides finding ways of dealing with the illness, things that can help you and your loved one to survive the bipolar disorder and enjoy your relationship and lives include:

- doing things you enjoy together
- relating to the person behind the illness and the things you like about each other, for example, their sense of humour, kindness, quick wit and creativity
- slowly rebuilding intimacy
- taking time and space to develop your own lives
- being mutually supportive
- encouraging each other's abilities and strengths and ways of expressing them while managing the illness

- using the communication skills mentioned in chapter 19 to maintain your relationship.

KEY POINTS

- Bipolar disorder affects the lives of close relatives and friends of the person with the illness. Not all people who care for someone with bipolar disorder are affected in the same way.
- The changes resulting from bipolar disorder include the challenges presented by difficult symptoms and extra demands. They may affect work and social life as well as financial security.
- Emotional and sexual intimacy may suffer, and you may experience many strong and difficult emotions and even become depressed.
- Helpful ways of coping include knowing about the illness, its causes and treatment, coming to terms with it, maintaining your boundaries and your life, and developing collaborative plans to make the illness more manageable.
- You can move beyond blame and guilt to understanding the complicated nature of bipolar disorder, and having realistic expectations for yourself and others about managing it.
- Meanwhile, there is a lot you can do to enjoy and sustain your relationship.
- The experiences of people who care for someone with bipolar disorder vary greatly, and you need to find what works for you.

GLOSSARY

Anxiety disorders A category of mental illness that is characterised by such feelings as fear, worry or apprehension. Anxiety disorders include social phobia, agoraphobia, panic attacks, generalised anxiety disorder, phobias, and post-traumatic stress disorder.

Anxiolytic Medication used to treat symptoms of anxiety.

Atypical antipsychotics A newer type of antipsychotic with fewer side effects, used to treat bipolar disorder.

Atypical depression Refers to a particular set of symptoms that occurs with a major depressive or dysthymic episode. With atypical depression a person experiences increased appetite, excessive sleep, lethargy or fatigue, and may be sensitive to being rejected.

Bipolar I A category of bipolar disorder characterised by episodes of mania. People with this type of bipolar disorder may or may not also experience periods of depression.

Bipolar II A category of bipolar disorder characterised by episodes of hypomania and depression.

Bipolar not otherwise specified (NOS) A category of bipolar disorder where the symptoms do not meet all the criteria for bipolar disorder, but where bipolar disorder features are clearly present.

Bipolar spectrum This term is often used to refer to the bipolar diagnostic categories of bipolar I, bipolar II and cyclothymia, as listed in the DSM-IV. It has also been used more broadly to include periods of elevated mood, which currently do not meet the criteria of the current diagnostic system (DSM).

Blunted A reduction or lack of emotional intensity.

Breakthrough episodes Episodes of illness which occur despite taking medication.

Chronic illness A long-lasting or recurrent illness.

Cognitive behavioural therapy A form of psychotherapy that focuses on unhelpful thoughts and behaviours.

Cognitive therapy A form of psychotherapy that focuses on unhelpful thoughts.

Comorbidity Experiencing two or more disorders (diagnoses) at the same time, for example bipolar disorder and social phobia.

Combination therapy The use of more than one medication to treat a disorder.

Coping skill A tool or strategy to better manage a situation or event.

Cyclothymia A pattern of fluctuating mood involving hypo-manic symptoms and depressive symptoms, which do not meet the full criteria for a diagnosis of depression. Symptom-free periods last less than two months and the general mood fluctuations last at least two years.

Delusion A false belief regarding the self or persons or objects outside the self that persists despite the facts, and occurs in some psychotic states.

Diagnosis The identification of a disease or disorder, based on a series of symptoms and signs, which accord with a particular disorder.

DSM-IV *Diagnostic and Statistical Manual of Mental Disorders,* (Fourth Edition), contains the diagnostic criteria for mental disorders. Published by the American Psychiatric Association, these diagnoses are agreed upon by international reference groups. The DSM-IV is a widely used international guide for clinicians.

Dysphoric mania Another term for mixed states or mixed mania.

Dysthymia Chronically lowered (depressed) mood for most of the time, most days. The symptoms are not as severe as in a depressive episode, but last for at least two years.

Electroconvulsive therapy A procedure in which an electrical current is briefly administered to the brain while the person is under a light general anaesthetic. Used to treat depression, mania and mixed episodes.

Family-focused therapy A form of psychotherapy that involves the whole family. Components include education, communication and problem solving.

Flatness Refers to an emotional state where the person displays a lack of interest or animation in things.

Hallucination Perception of something (as a visual image or a sound) with no external cause, usually arising from a disorder of the nervous system.

Homeostasis The property of a living organism to regulate its internal environment so as to maintain a stable, constant condition.

Hormones Circulating chemicals that transmit messages to internal organs, e.g. cortisol, thyroid hormone.

Hypnotics Medications used to treat insomnia.

Hypomania A period of constant elevated or irritable mood lasting at least four days that is not as severe or disruptive as mania.

Interpersonal and social rhythm therapy This therapy explores the role of illness on a person's life and monitors social rhythms such as sleep/wake cycle and activity level.

Labile moods Quickly changing moods.

Life chart A life chart records episodes of illness and wellness over time, with corresponding life events. It is used to assist in the identification of personal triggers.

Maintenance treatment Ongoing treatment designed to reduce the recurrence of an episode of illness.

Major depression Significantly lowered mood and/or a loss of interest or pleasure in things, plus at least five other symptoms of lowered mood, that lasts at least two weeks and affects your daily life.

Mania An abnormally elevated or irritable mood, plus at least three or four other symptoms of mania, that lasts at least a week and affects your daily life.

Mindfulness-based cognitive therapy A form of therapy initially used in treatment of stress and chronic pain. This approach teaches the recognition and acceptance of thoughts and feelings and of just 'being' rather than reacting and 'doing'.

Mixed episodes Refers to the occurrence of both a manic and a depressive episode at the same time. To meet diagnostic criteria for this category the symptoms need to be present for at least a week.

Mixed depression When symptoms of mania are present in an episode of depression.

Mood A conscious state of mind that lasts longer than a fleeting emotion and includes feelings, thoughts and behaviour.

Mood stabilisers A medication that can prevent new episodes of either depression or mania.

Poles Refers to the two types of bipolar episode, the elevated (manic) pole and the lowered (depressed) pole.

Prodromes Early signs or symptoms indicating that an episode of illness may be imminent.

Psychoeducation Education about an illness combined with information on helpful management strategies.

Psychotherapy Refers to a range of techniques and processes between a registered practitioner and client to address a diversity of issues, which may relate to a mental illness, emotional difficulties, or issues regarding problems of daily life and relationships.

Psychotic symptoms Symptoms that reflect a loss of contact with reality, such as hallucinations or delusions. These might include disordered thinking, beliefs about being followed or persecuted, or having special powers or abilities.

Relapse A recurrence of an episode of illness.

Relapse signature An individual's personal warning signs of illness.

Rapid cycling Refers to the rapid recurrence of episodes of illness. Official criteria suggest there must be at least four episodes of illness in a one-year period.

Residual symptoms Refers to symptoms left over from episode of illness. These symptoms are not significant enough to constitute an episode of illness, but may cause interference with day-to-day life.

Schizophrenia A psychotic disorder characterised by a loss of contact with reality. This results in the experience of delusions and/or hallucinations, confused thoughts and speech, and unusual behaviour.

Schizoaffective disorder This disorder occurs when symptoms of a mood disorder (either depression, mania or a mixed episode) and schizophrenia occur together, but psychotic symptoms are present for at least two weeks without mood symptoms.

Self-management Refers to a process of gaining more control over the illness through having a personal understanding of the illness and using strategies to deal with it.

Subsyndromal symptoms Experiencing symptoms, but not enough for them to meet criteria for a full episode of illness.

Symptoms From the Latin *symptoma*, meaning 'chance, accident, mischance'. Symptom refers to a change from what is usual.

Symptomatic Showing signs of illness.

Temperament Aspects of general make-up or nature.

Trigger Something that brings about (triggers) an episode of illness.

Unipolar depression Depression that occurs without any history of episodes of mood elevation (such as mania or hypomania).

Warning symptoms Changes that indicate that an episode of illness is brewing (such as changes to usual sleep pattern).

BIBLIOGRAPHY

Abou-Saleh, M.T. & Coppen, A. (2006) Folic acid and the treatment of depression. *J Psychosom Res*, 61, 285–7.

Akiskal, H.S., Hantouche, E.G., Bourgeois, M.L., Azorin, J.M., Sechter, D., Allilaire, J.F., Lancrenon, S., Fraud, J.P. & Chatenet-Duchene, L. (1998) Gender, temperament, and the clinical picture in dysphoric mixed mania: findings from a French national study (EPIMAN). *J Affect Disord*, 50, 175–86.

American Psychiatric Association (2000) *Diagnostic and statistical manual of mental disorders*, Washington DC, American Psychiatric Association.

Anthony, W.A. (1993) Recovering from mental illness: the guiding vision of the mental health service system in the 1990s. *Psychosocial Rehabilitation Journal*, 16, 11–23.

Bachmann, R.F., Schloesser, R.J., Gould, T.D. & Manji, H.K. (2005) Mood stabilizers target cellular plasticity and resilience cascades: implications for the development of novel therapeutics. *Mol Neurobiol*, 32, 173–202.

Balázs, J., Benazzi, F., Rihmer, Z., Rihmer, A., Akiskal, K.K. & Akiskal, H.S. (2006) The close link between suicide attempts and mixed (bipolar) depression: implications for suicide prevention. *J Affect Disord*, 91, 133–8.

Basco, M. (2006) *The bipolar workbook: tools for controlling your moodswings*, New York, Guilford Press.

Bauer, M.S. & McBride, L. (2003) *Structured group psychotherapy for bipolar disorder: the life goals program*, New York, Springer Pub.

Benazzi, F. (2007) Bipolar disorder—focus on bipolar II disorder and mixed depression. *Lancet*, 369, 935–45.

Berk, M., Berk, L., Castle, D. (2004) A collaborative approach to the treatment alliance in bipolar disorder. *Bipolar Disorders*, 6, 504–18.

Berk, M. (2007) Should we be targeting smoking as a routine intervention? *Acta Neuropsychiatrica*, 19, 131–132.

Brady, K.T. & Sonne, S.C. (1995) The relationship between substance abuse and bipolar disorder. *J Clin Psychiatry*, 56 Suppl 3, 19–24.

Brunello, N. & Tascedda, F. (2003) Cellular mechanisms and second messengers: relevance to the psychopharmacology of bipolar disorders. *Int J Neuropsychopharmacol*, 6, 181–9.

Cassidy, F., Ahearn, E., Murry, E., Forest, K. & Carroll, B.J. (2000) Diagnostic depressive symptoms of the mixed bipolar episode. *Psychol Med*, 30, 403–11.

Castle, D., Berk, M., Berk, L., Lauder, S., Chamberlain, J. & Gilbert, M. Pilot of group intervention for bipolar disorder. *Int J Psychiat Clin*, In Press.

Chang, K., Karchemskiy, A., Barnea-Goraly, N., Garrett, A., Simeonova, D.I. & Reiss, A. (2005) Reduced amygdala gray matter volume in familial paediatric bipolar disorder. *J Am Acad Child Adolesc Psychiatry*, 44, 565–73.

Colom, F. & Vieta, E. (2006) *Manual for bipolar disorder*, Cambridge University Press.

Colom, F., Vieta, E., Martinez-Aran, A., Reinares, M., Goikolea, J.M., Benabarre, A., Torrent, C., Comes, M., Corbella, B., Parramon, G. & Corominas, J. (2003a) A randomized trial on the efficacy of group psychoeducation in the prophylaxis of recurrences in bipolar patients whose disease is in remission. *Arch Gen Psychiatry*, 60, 402–7.

Colom, F., Vieta, E., Reinares, M., Martinez-Aran, A., Torrent, C., Goikolea, J.M. & Gasto, C. (2003b) Psychoeducation efficacy in bipolar disorders: beyond compliance enhancement. *J Clin Psychiatry*, 64, 1101–5.

Cuellar, A.K., Johnson, S.L. & Winters, R. (2005) Distinctions between bipolar and unipolar depression. *Clin Psychol Rev*, 25, 307–39.

De Hert, M., Thys, E., Magiels, G. & Wyckaert, S. (2004) *Anything or nothing: self guide for people with bipolar disorder*, Antwerp, Uitgeverij Houtekiet.

Deegan, P.E. (1994) 'Recovery: the lived experience of rehabilitation' in *Readings in psychiatric rehabilitation*, W.A. Anthony & I. Spaniol (eds), pp. 142–62, Boston, Boston University, Centre for Psychiatric Rehabilitation.

Dore, G. & Romans, S.E. (2001) Impact of bipolar affective disorder on family and partners. *J Affect Disord*, 67, 147–58.

Dumville, J.C., Miles, J.N., Porthouse, J., Cockayne, S., Saxon, L. & King, C. (2006) Can vitamin D supplementation prevent winter-time blues? A randomised trial among older women. *J Nutr Health Aging*, 10, 151–3.

Edelman, S. (2002) *Change your thinking: positive and practical ways to overcome stress, negative emotions and self-defeating behaviour using CBT*, Sydney, ABC Books for the Australian Broadcasting Corporation.

Erman, M. (2005) Therapeutic options in the treatment of insomnia. *J Clin Psychiatry*, 66, 18–23.

Fast, J.A. & Preston, J. (2004) *Loving someone with bipolar disorder: understanding and helping your partner*, Canada, London, New Harbinger, Hi Marketing.

Frank, E. (2007) Interpersonal and social rhythm therapy: a means of improving depression and preventing relapse in bipolar disorder. *J Clin Psychol*, 63, 463–73.

Gibran, K. (1980) *The prophet* [1923], London, Heinemann: distributed by Pan Books.

Gilbert, P. (2000) *Overcoming depression*, London, Robinson.

Goodwin, F.K. & Jamison, K.R. (1990) *Manic-depressive illness*, New York, Oxford University Press.

Goodwin, F. & Redfield Jamison, K. (2007) *Manic-depressive illness*, New York, Oxford University Press.

Greenberger, D. & Padesky, C. (1995) *Mind over mood: change how you feel by changing the way you think*, New York, Guildford Press.

Hallam, K.T., Olver, J.S., Chambers, V., Begg, D.P., McGrath, C. & Norman, T.R. (2006) The heritability of melatonin secretion and sensitivity to bright nocturnal light in twins. *Psychoneuroendocrinology*, 31, 867–75.

Harris, E.C. & Barraclough, B. (1997) Suicide as an outcome for mental disorders: a meta-analysis. *Br J Psychiatry*, 170, 205–28.

Hayes, S.C. & Smith, S.X. (2005) *Get out of your mind and into your life: the new acceptance and commitment therapy*, Oakland, CA, New Harbinger Publications.

Hirschfeld, R., Lewis, L. & Vornik, L. (2003) Perceptions and impact of bipolar disorder: how far have we really come? Results of the National Depressive and Manic-Depressive Association 2000 survey of individuals with bipolar disorder. *J Clin Psychiatry*, 64, 161–74.

Jamison, K.R. (1997) *An unquiet mind*, London, A.A. Knopf.

Johnson, L., Lundstrom, O., Aberg-Wistedt, A. & Mathe, A.A. (2003) Social support in bipolar disorder: its relevance to remission and relapse. *Bipolar Disord*, 5, 129–37.

Johnson, S.L. (2005) Life events in bipolar disorder: towards more specific models. *Clin Psychol Rev*, 25, 1008–27.

Johnson, S.L., Meyer, B., Winett, C. & Small, J. (2000) Social support and self-esteem predict changes in bipolar depression but not mania. *J Affect Disord*, 58, 79–86.

Johnson, S.L., Winett, C.A., Meyer, B., Greenhouse, W.J. & Miller, I. (1999) Social support and the course of bipolar disorder. *J Abnorm Psychol*, 108, 558–66.

Jones, S., Hayward, P. & Lam, D. (2003) *Coping with bipolar disorder*, Oxford, Oneworld Publications.

Kabat-Zinn, J. (1990) *Full catastrophe living: using the wisdom of your body and mind to face stress, pain, and illness*, New York, Delacorte Press.

Kelly, M. (2000) *Life on a roller coaster: living well with depression and manic depression*, Australia, Simon & Schuster.

Kelsoe, J.R. & Niculescu, A.B., III (2002) Finding genes for bipolar disorder in the functional genomics era: from convergent functional genomics to phonemics and back. *CNS Spectr*, 7, 215–6, 223–6.

Lam, D. & Wong, G. (1997) Prodromes, coping strategies, insight and social functioning in bipolar affective disorders. *Psychol Med*, 27, 1091–100.

Lam, D. & Wong, G. (2006) 'Bipolar relapse: the importance of early warning signs and coping strategies' in *The psychology of bipolar disorder: new developments and research strategies*, S.H. Jones and R.P. Bentall (eds), New York, Oxford University Press.

Lam, D., Wong, G. & Sham, P. (2001) Prodromes, coping strategies and course of illness in bipolar affective disorder—a naturalistic study. *Psychol Med*, 31, 1397–402.

Lam, D.H., Watkins, E.R., Hayward, P., Bright, J., Wright, K., Kerr, N., Parr-Davis, G. & Sham, P. (2003) A randomized controlled study of cognitive therapy for relapse prevention for bipolar affective disorder: outcome of the first year. *Arch Gen Psychiatry*, 60, 145–52.

Leibenluft, E. & Suppes, T. (1999) Treating bipolar illness: focus on treatment algorithms and management of the sleep-wake cycle. *Am J Psychiatry*, 156, 1976–81.

Lewis, L. & Hoofnagle, L. (2005) Patient perspectives on provider competence: a view from the Depression and Bipolar Support Alliance. *Adm Policy Ment Health*, 32, 497–503.

Linehan, M. (1993) *Cognitive-behavioural treatment of borderline personality disorder*, New York, Guilford Press.

Linehan, M.M., Goodstein, J.L., Nielsen, S.L. & Chiles, J.A. (1983) Reasons for staying alive when you are thinking of killing yourself: the reasons for living inventory. *J Consult Clin Psychol*, 51, 276–86.

Marra, T. (2004) *Depressed and anxious: the dialectical behaviour therapy workbook for overcoming depression and anxiety*, Oakland, CA, New Harbinger.

McIntyre, R.S., Soczynska, J.K., Bottas, A., Bordbar, K., Konarski, J.Z. & Kennedy, S.H. (2006) Anxiety disorders and bipolar disorder: a review. *Bipolar Disord*, 8, 665–76.

McManamy, J. (2006) *Living well with depression and bipolar disorder: what your doctor doesn't tell you . . . that you need to know*, New York, HarperCollins.

Michalak, E.E., Yatham, L.N., Kolesar, S. & Lam, R.W. (2006) Bipolar disorder and quality of life: a patient-centered perspective. *Qual Life Res*, 15, 25–37.

Miklowitz, D.J. (2002) *The bipolar disorder survival guide*, New York, The Guilford Press.

Miklowitz, D.J., Goldstein, M.J., Nuechterlein, K.H., Snyder, K.S. & Mintz, J. (1988) Family factors and the course of bipolar affective disorder. *Arch Gen Psychiatry*, 45, 225–31.

Miklowitz, D.J., George, J.A., Richards, T.L., et al. (2003). A randomised study of family-focused psychoeducation and pharmacotherapy in the outpatient management of bipolar disorder. *Arch Gen Psychiatry*, 60(9), 904–912.

Molnar, G., Feeney, M.G. & Fava, G.A. (1988) Duration and symptoms of bipolar prodromes. *Am J Psychiatry*, 145, 1576–8.

Newman, C., Leahy, R.L., Beck, A.T., Reilly-Harrington, N.A. & Gyulai, L. (2002) *Bipolar disorder: a cognitive therapy approach*, Washington DC, American Psychological Association.

Ng, F., Dodd, S. & Berk, M. (2007) The effects of physical activity in the acute treatment of bipolar disorder: a pilot study. *Journal of Affective Disorders*, 101, 259–62.

Oliwenstein, L. (2004) *Taming bipolar disorder*, USA, Alpha Books.

Perlick, D.A., Rosenheck, R.A., Clarkin, J.F., Maciejewski, P.K., Sirey, J., Struening, E. & Link, B.G. (2004) Impact of family burden and affective response on clinical outcome among patients with bipolar disorder. *Psychiatr Serv*, 55, 1029–35.

Perlis, R.H., Ostacher, M.J., Patel, J.K., Marangell, L.B., Zhang, H., Wisniewski, S.R., Ketter, T.A., Miklowitz, D.J., Otto, M.W., Gyulai, L., Reilly-Harrington, N.A., Nierenberg, A.A., Sachs, G.S. & Thase, M.E. (2006) Predictors of recurrence in bipolar disorder: primary outcomes from the Systematic Treatment Enhancement Program for Bipolar Disorder (STEP-BD). *Am J Psychiatry*, 163, 217–24.

Perry, A., Tarrier, N., Morriss, R., McCarthy, E. & Limb, K. (1999) Randomised controlled trial of efficacy of teaching patients with bipolar disorder to identify early symptoms of relapse and obtain treatment. *BMJ*, 318, 149–53.

Potash, J.B. & DePaulo, J.R., Jr. (2000) Searching high and low: a review of the genetics of bipolar disorder. *Bipolar Disord*, 2, 8–26.

Reinares, M., Vieta, E., Colom, F., Martinez-Aran, A., Torrent, C., Comes, M., Goikolea, J.M., Benabarre, A., Daban, C. & Sanchez-Moreno, J. (2006) What really matters to bipolar patients' caregivers: sources of family burden. *J Affect Disord*, 94, 157–63.

Rihmer, Z. (2007) Suicide risk in mood disorders. *Current Opinion in Psychiatry*, 20, 17–22.

Russell, S. (2005) *A lifelong journey: staying well with manic depression/bipolar disorder*, Australia, Michelle Anderson Publishing Pty Ltd.

Sachs, G. (1993) Mood Chart, available at <www.manicdepressive.org> Boston, Harvard Bipolar Research Program.

Schou, M. (1997) Forty years of lithium treatment. *Arch Gen Psychiatry*, 54, 9–13; discussion 14–5.

Scott, J. (2001) *Overcoming mood swings*, London, Robinson.

Scott, J. & Colom, F. (2005) Psychosocial treatments for bipolar disorders. *Psychiatr Clin North Am*, 28, 371–84.

Segal, Z.V., Williams, J.M.G. & Teasdale, J.D. (2002) *Mindfulness-based cognitive therapy for depression: a new approach to preventing relapse*, New York, Guilford Press.

Simon, G.E., Ludman, E.J., Bauer, M.S., Unutzer, J. & Operskalski, B. (2006) Long-term effectiveness and cost of a systematic care program for bipolar disorder. *Arch Gen Psychiatry*, 63, 500–8.

Singh, J.B. & Zarate, C.A., Jr. (2006) Pharmacological treatment of psychiatric comorbidity in bipolar disorder: a review of controlled trials. *Bipolar Disord*, 8, 696–709.

Singh, N., Clements, K. & Singh, M. (2001) The efficacy of exercise as a long term antidepressant in elderly subjects: a randomized controlled trial. *Journal of Gerontology*, 56.

Smoller, J.W. & Finn, C.T. (2003) Family, twin, and adoption studies of bipolar disorder. *Am J Med Genet C Semin Med Genet*, 123, 48–58.

Sontrop, J. & Campbell, M.K. (2006) Omega-3 polyunsaturated fatty acids and depression: a review of the evidence and a methodological critique. *Prev Med*, 42, 4–13.

Spence, J., McGannon, K. & Poon, P. (2005) The effect of exercise on global self esteem. A quantitative review. *J Sport and Exercise Psychology*, 27, 311–34.

Tanner, S. & Ball, J. (1999) *Beating the blues: a self-help approach to overcoming depression*, Sydney, Doubleday.

Thakore, J.H. & Dinan, T.G. (1996) Blunted dexamethasone-induced growth hormone responses in acute mania. *Psychoneuroendocrinology*, 21, 695–701.

Tondo, L. & Baldessarini, R.J. (2000) Reduced suicide risk during lithium maintenance treatment. *J Clin Psychiatry*, 61 Suppl 9, 97–104.

Wadee, A.A., Kuschke, R.H., Wood, L.A., Berk, M., Ichim, L. & Maes, M. (2002) Serological observations in patients suffering from acute manic episodes. *Hum Psychopharmacol*, 17, 175–9.

Woolis, R. (2003) *When someone you love has a mental illness: a handbook for family, friends, and caregivers*, New York, Jeremy P. Tarcher/Putnam.

World Health Organisation (2006) *Pocket guide to the ICD-10 classification of mental and behavioural disorders*, Geneva, Churchill Livingstone.

Yapko, M.D. (1997) *Breaking the patterns of depression*, New York, Doubleday.

Yin, L., Wang, J., Klein, P.S. & Lazar, M.A. (2006) Nuclear receptor Rev-erb alpha is a critical lithium-sensitive component of the circadian clock. *Science*, 311, 1002–5.

Young, S.L. & Ensing, D.S. (1999) Exploring recovery from the perspective of people with psychiatric disabilities. *Psychiatr Rehabil J*, 22, 219–231.

INDEX

Also available from Vermilion

The Devil Within

by Stephanie Merritt

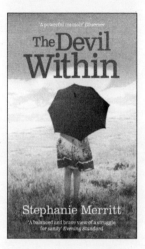

Stephanie Merritt has a career as a novelist and journalist, a beautiful son and a supportive family. Why then did she want to kill herself at the age of 29? Why could no one, neither the system of GPs and health professionals, nor her closest family and friends help her?

Beautifully written and intensely honest this is an extraordinarily moving, life-affirming book about a debilitating illness that affects one in six people in the UK alone. Reading like a hybrid of Elizabeth Wurtzel's *Prozac Nation* and Rachel Cusk's more sober *A Life's Work*, this is Stephanie's unflinchingly honest memoir of her experience with depression.

£7.99   ISBN 9780091917463   www.rbooks.co.uk

Trouble in My Head

by Mathilde Monaque

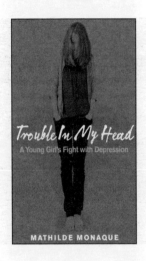

Mathilde Monaque developed severe depression when she was just 14. The eldest in a family of six and an exceptionally bright and gifted little girl, the discovery shook her family to the core.

Trouble in My Head is Mathilde's tender and illuminating account of her struggle to surface from a disease that could have taken her life. With remarkable sensitivity and lucidity she describes her unique experience of teenage depression. Unlike adult depression, which involves feelings of guilt, Mathilde describes teenage depression as a breaking down of certainties, the fear of being oneself, the fear of not loving and of not being loved.

Adults and teenagers alike will find inspiration and insight in her touching and remarkable account.

£8.99   ISBN 9780091917234   www.rbooks.co.uk

10 Days to Great Self Esteem

by David Burns

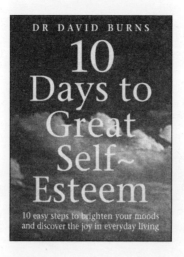

Do you wake up dreading the day? Do you feel discouraged with what you've accomplished in life? Do you want greater self-esteem, productivity, and joy in daily living?

In *10 Days to Great Self Esteem*, Dr David Burns offers a powerful tool providing hope, compassion, and healing for people suffering from low self-esteem or unhappiness. In ten easy steps you will learn specific techniques to enhance self esteem, productivity and happiness. With ideas based on commonsense and easy to apply, Dr Burns helps you feel the way you think and change the way you feel brightening your outlook when you're in a slump for happier everyday living.

£11.99   ISBN 9780091825621   www.rbooks.co.uk

FREE POSTAGE AND PACKING

Overseas customers allow £2.00 per paperback

BY PHONE: 01624 677237

BY POST: Random House Books
C/o Bookpost, PO Box 29, Douglas
Isle of Man, IM99 1BQ

BY FAX: 01624 670923

BY EMAIL: bookshop@enterprise.net

Cheques (payable to Bookpost) and credit cards accepted

Prices and availability subject to change without notice.
Allow 28 days for delivery.
When placing your order, please mention if you do not
wish to receive any additional information.

www.rbooks.co.uk